MY JOURNEY WITH NEUROENDOCRINE CANCER

What You Don't Know Can Kill You!

By Bob Walsh

BOB WALSH

MY JOURNEY WITH NEUROENDOCRINE CANCER
What You Don't Know Can Kill You!

MY JOURNEY WITH NEUROENDOCRINE CANCER
What You Don't Know Can Kill You!

With the exception of short excerpts for critical reviews, no part of this book may be reproduced or transmitted in any form or by any means, electronic, mechanical or otherwise including photocopying, recording, or any information storage or retrieval system, without the express permission in writing from the author, except as provided by United States of America Copyright Law.

© Copyright Pending 2018 by Robert T. Walsh
With the Library of Congress
All rights reserved.

Paperback ISBN: 9781731022134
Cover design and photos by Bob Walsh
Editing by Margie Holly Walsh

Published by PBJ Enterprises, Inc.
162 Liberty Street, Deer Park, New York 11729
United States of America
Email: walsh516@aol.com

Printed and bound in the United States of America
First Edition

BOB WALSH

MY JOURNEY WITH NEUROENDOCRINE CANCER
What You Don't Know Can Kill You!

CONTENTS

Dedication		vii
About the Author		ix
Author's Notes		xiii
Preface		xv

SECTION ONE - MY JOURNEY

Chapter 1	My NET Cancer Nightmare Begins	01
Chapter 2	"There's Bleeding Inside Your Eye"	07
Chapter 3	"A Tumor Is Blocking Everything!"	11
Chapter 4	"There's More Bleeding in Your Eye!"	15
Chapter 5	Becoming a "Zebra"	19
Chapter 6	"You Need the Whipple!"	23
Chapter 7	Miracle at Saint Anne's Shrine in NYC	29
Chapter 8	"I Have Other Patients with Real Cancer!"	35
Chapter 9	Doctor Edward Wolin	43
Chapter 10	"The Tumor is Gone!"	47
Chapter 11	"We May Not be Able to Save Your Sight!"	51
Chapter 12	National Institutes of Health (NIH)	53
Chapter 13	"A Definite Maybe"	61
Chapter 14	Doctor Grossly Inept	63
Chapter 15	NIH's Surgical Knight in Armor	71
Chapter 16	Trying to Save My Sight	75
Chapter 17	"You Look So Good!"	77
Chapter 18	The "Wait and See" Treatment Plan	79
Chapter 19	The Sight in My Right Eye is Gone!	81
Chapter 20	Doctor Grossly Inept Strikes Again!	83
Chapter 21	St. Elizabeth's Parish	85
Chapter 22	Mishaps at NIH	87
Chapter 23	Doctor Grossly Inept Cripples Me!	99
Chapter 24	"Doctor Pain"	105
Chapter 25	The Dreaded Three Inch Needle	107
Chapter 26	Blood Tests Alone Can Miss NET Cancer!	111

Chapter 27	"You May Never Fully Heal"	113
Chapter 28	Doctor Pain Tries to Help	115
Chapter 29	Needle Biopsy of My Thyroid	117
Chapter 30	A Second Killer NET Tumor Appears!	121
Chapter 31	God Does It Again - A Second Miracle!	131
Chapter 32	The Greatest Medicine of All	133

SECTION TWO - TECHNICAL REFERENCES

Chapter 33	The Neuroendocrine System	137
Chapter 34	Neuroendocrine Cancer	139
Chapter 35	Carcinoid Tumors	147
Chapter 36	Types of Neuroendocrine Tumors (NETs)	149
Chapter 37	Symptoms of Neuroendocrine Cancer	155
Chapter 38	The Carcinoid Syndrome	163
Chapter 39	Carcinoid Crisis	165
Chapter 40	Treating Neuroendocrine Cancer	167
Chapter 41	Peptide Receptor Radionuclide Therapy	175
Chapter 42	Information Resources on the Internet	181
Chapter 43	Glossary of Neuroendocrine Cancer Terms	191

EXHIBITS

A	Letter to Local Clergy Regarding Recent Miracles	201
B	Biopsy Pathology Report Shows 1st NET Tumor	204
C	Biopsy Pathology Report Shows 1st Tumor Disappears	205
D	CT/PET Scan Report Shows 2nd NET Tumor	206
E	Biopsy Pathology Report Shows 2nd Tumor Disappears	207

Select Books Published by PBJ Enterprises, Inc.	209
Index	213
Notes	217

MY JOURNEY WITH NEUROENDOCRINE CANCER
What You Don't Know Can Kill You!

DEDICATION

This book is dedicated to all the wonderful people who have assisted me on my difficult journey with neuroendocrine cancer. Often called "NET Cancer" by patients, this is considered one of the rarest, little understood cancers of them all.

In particular, I extend my love and deep appreciation to my wife, Margie Holly Walsh, ever loving and encouraging, she has stood by my side throughout my struggles with this terrible cancer.

Special thanks go to my younger sister, Diana Walsh, a fellow NET cancer survivor herself, diagnosed shortly before I learned I also had it. Yes, oncologists have clinically confirmed that neuroendocrine cancer has been found to run in families. Diana provided me with valuable information on this rare cancer and referred me to the few doctors and oncologists familiar with neuroendocrine cancer.

My gratitude goes as well to the medical professionals who give cancer patients like me a fighting chance to battle this dread disease and possibly outlive it.

BOB WALSH

MY JOURNEY WITH NEUROENDOCRINE CANCER
What You Don't Know Can Kill You!

ABOUT THE AUTHOR
Bob Walsh

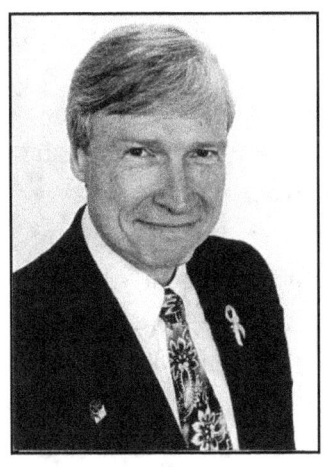

One of 12 children, I grew up in a small, four room apartment in the Yorkville section on the east side of Manhattan in the heart of New York City during the 1940s and 50s. I married my teenage sweetheart, Margie Holly, and together we raised our three children while I worked as a bank executive on Wall Street. When my parents died at an early age, Margie and I also cared for four of my younger sisters.

Following a career on Wall Street, I briefly served as a U.S. Goodwill Ambassador to Russia and Ukraine, was a candidate for Governor of New York in 1994 and for U.S. Congress in 2000.

In my parish of Ss. Cyril and Methodius in Deer Park, Long Island, New York, I have served as a Catholic Eucharistic Minister since 1978, have been a member of the Holy Name Society, Knights of Columbus and served as a Confirmation Catechist. Since 2013, I have written and published several business and religious books distributed online worldwide.

In 2009, I was diagnosed with two different types of malignant cancer -prostate cancer and a rare form of malignant skin cancer. I survived extensive surgeries to remove these deadly malignancies without chemo or radiation. Around the same time, I also learned that I had Hemochromatosis (often referred to as "iron-overload"). Since this condition can be fatal unless a pint of blood is withdrawn on a regular basis, I have this done every two months.

In early 2017, I was diagnosed with neuroendocrine cancer ... another type of malignant cancer. Often called "NET cancer" by patients, I discovered there was relatively little information and understanding for this rare, deadly cancer. As you will read, just when it appeared one of the tumors was going to end my life, an utterly remarkable miracle occurred. God took the deadly tumor away ... but not the cancer!

Given all physical biopsies, scans and other medical evidence clearly, irrefutably showing the presence of the malignant tumor in me, all the doctors and oncologists were at a loss to explain how this tumor could possibly disappear. In fact, six leading oncology research centers in America subsequently have examined all the medical evidence and concurred ... there is no earthly way to scientifically explain how this happened.

My wife, Margie, and I confidently told everyone that God had interceded in answer to the countless prayers and Masses said on my behalf. Some of the dedicated oncologists and research professionals specializing in this rare cancer agreed with us ... but most did not. So many just could not accept the possibility that something so miraculous, so inexplicable could happen in a case involving such an incurable, deadly malignancy.

Perhaps it was for very reason that God interceded a second time! A little over a year later in late 2018, another lethal NET tumor never seen before suddenly appeared and clearly identified! Like the first one a year earlier, this tumor was located in my digestive system at virtually the same place as the tumor that miraculously disappeared.

This time, I went to a different leading oncology center that also specialized in the research and treatment of neuroendocrine cancer, Mount Sinai Hospital in New York City. This was to be the seventh such major oncology center in America to treat me for this rare cancer. These oncologists had previously heard much about me since I had the rarest of the rare NET cancer – and they were well aware of the reported miraculous disappearance of the first tumor.

MY JOURNEY WITH NEUROENDOCRINE CANCER
What You Don't Know Can Kill You!

However scientifically curious and skeptical they were, that did not last too long. Right before the eyes of some of the very best oncologists in the world, God interceded again! For a second time, He miraculously removed the new entrenched tumor - in exactly same way and manner He did a year before! God has given everyone - doctors and patients alike - a second utterly remarkable, miraculous event supported by clear, extensive scientific evidence.

It was then that I decided to write this book to share my experiences battling this rare cancer, and what I learned about it. Most importantly, it was also to encourage everyone to trust God, strong in faith and include Him in all things.

73 years of life have taught me one clear, undeniable truth. The very best way to enjoy all the good things of life - and to deal with the inevitable painful, dark times that come to all of us - is to keep God in our hearts and minds ... and to allow His words in holy scripture to guide us in all things.

As a personal witness to the miraculous, my hope in sharing my journey is that it may provide some helpful information and encouragement for fellow cancer patients, their caregivers, doctors and oncologists, and for future generations in my circle of family and friends.

With God leading the way, I know our very best days are yet to come. I truly pray that God will guide you and bless you, my reader, and all those you carry in your heart, as we all travel on the most important journey of all - the one that leads to Heaven.

BOB WALSH

AUTHOR'S NOTES

Much of the information presented in this book was found through various Internet resources you can find listed in one of my last chapters. The material provided does not endorse nor does it recommend any doctor, oncologist, medical facility, medication or treatment plan. In all cases, readers are encouraged to seek the advice and guidance of healthcare professionals when dealing with health issues. Most importantly, wherever your journey in life may take you, make sure to include God in all you do.

BOB WALSH

MY JOURNEY WITH NEUROENDOCRINE CANCER
What You Don't Know Can Kill You!

PREFACE

In early 2017, I was surprised to learn I had something in common with a number of well-known celebrities including John Wayne, Betty Davis, Aretha Franklin, Steve Jobs and the great NFL running back, Walter Payton. What we all had in common was a very rare cancer by the name of neuroendocrine cancer.

With no warning, in late February 2017, I learned I had this rare, incurable malignancy. This news shook me to my very core since I had already previously struggled with and survived two other deadly malignancies - prostate cancer and a rare form of highly malignant skin cancer.

Like other cancer patients receiving such devastating news, a tsunami of troublesome thoughts swept through my mind every day and night. "What is this cancer all about? Is it going to kill me? How is it that none of my doctors and oncologists treating me over the years never detected the presence of THIS cancer?"

These thoughts hounded me and were followed by other tormenting questions. "Does this cancer have anything to do with the other two malignancies I've had? How much time do I have? How do I fight this cancer? Am I going to suffer badly? Will I have to go through surgery, chemo and/or radiation? How do I tell my family and friends? If I am going to die, how will my wife and family manage without me?"

Ultimately, these worrisome thoughts were replaced with a combative determination to battle this newest cancer and survive it. "I am going to fight this cancer, and I am **NOT** going to allow it to destroy the quality of my life ... and that of my family and friends!"

My thoughts soon evolved to wonder if this neuroendocrine cancer had anything to do with the many years of physical suffering I had endured with unexplained, painful conditions. As the pieces gradually fell into place, the answer was a resounding yes!

Neuroendocrine cancer contributed, in part, to the extraordinary, mysterious pains and sufferings I had experienced most of my life.

My focus quickly turned to determining what I could to do to fight this deadly cancer. The first challenge was, in fact, to learn everything I could about this monster that was living and growing inside me. I soon learned, however, it was very difficult to locate much clear, meaningful information on neuroendocrine cancer. Worse yet, I also discovered it was nearly impossible to find a medical doctor or oncologist with an understanding of this deadly cancer! As this reality set in, a shroud of fear descended upon me.

"What am I to do?" I remember lamenting at the time. "God help me."

It was bad enough I had this highly rare, sinister, mysterious malignancy, but then I had to deal with so many physicians and oncologists who were not familiar with it. Realizing I was in the fight of my life to survive, I felt as if I was blindfolded, stumbling on a long, unfamiliar road with a monstrous cancer creature stalking me ... intent on overcoming and destroying me. I felt like David against Goliath, and could imagine how St. Peter must have felt as he walked on the water in the midst of a terrible storm at sea.

All this brought me to my knees as I cried out to God for help. As a devout Catholic all my life, I found great comfort and solace in praying the rosary, attending Confession, Mass and Holy Communion.

As news of my dilemma quickly spread, family and friends prayed the rosary for me and offered countless Masses on my behalf. Spiritually strengthened, I set about doing battle with the deadly monster of neuroendocrine cancer. The more I learned about neuroendocrine cancer, the more hopeful and less helpless I felt. I found the sayings, "knowledge is power," and "knowing the enemy is half the battle," were so true.

Along the way I also heard how many of us NET cancer

MY JOURNEY WITH NEUROENDOCRINE CANCER
What You Don't Know Can Kill You!

patients suffer needlessly due to misinformation, misdiagnosis, lack of treatment and at times, outright mistreatment. In time, I was to personally suffer each of these during my own painful journey.

In writing this book, my hope is that fellow cancer patients, family and friends, caregivers, doctors and oncologists will find some hope and encouragement along with helpful facts, information and references to help in the battle with cancer.

May God bless you and all your loved ones with His love, peace, serenity and healing of mind, body and spirit. With God leading the way, our very best days are yet to come. I hope to see you all in Heaven some bright, glorious day.

BOB WALSH

MY JOURNEY WITH NEUROENDOCRINE CANCER
What You Don't Know Can Kill You!

SECTION ONE – MY JOURNEY

Chapter 1

MY NET CANCER NIGHTMARE BEGINS

During the early evening hours of Friday, February 10, 2017, I was relaxing at home in Deer Park, Long Island with my wife, Margie, and family members when an excruciating, crippling pain gripped the front-center of my torso. The agonizing pain was so severe, it effectively paralyzed me as I sat in a living room recliner. I was barely able to breathe.

As the merciless pain continued without pause, I began to shake and became violently ill with chills, nausea, fever and lethargy. I was so weak and crippled with pain, I could barely talk. Family members thought I might be having a heart attack so they wanted to take me to the hospital but I adamantly refused.

I assured everyone, "I know the pain doesn't involve my heart, it's coming from around my stomach. I have had this kind of pain before ... only not this bad. The 'cramps' should stop soon."

I had endured similar, excruciating attacks a number of times over the past few years. This time, however, the pains did not stop ... they continued unabated for several hours. I now realize how foolish and irresponsible it was for me to refuse to go to the emergency room of our local hospital located only fifteen minutes away. I could have died as the excruciating pain continued throughout the evening into the early morning hours.

During the night, my thoughts drifted back to a time earlier that week when I went to see my primary care physician, Dr. Howard Hertz, at his office on Main Street in Babylon, Long Island. Dr. Hertz was highly regarded by many in our local community including several doctors who used Dr. Hertz as their own primary care physician.

I sought his medical advice at the time since my regularly scheduled phlebotomy (bloodletting) once every eight weeks was not allowed by a doctor at the Greater New York Blood Center in Huntington, Long Island, New York. He said the hematocrit level of my blood was well below the minimum acceptable level for having a phlebotomy. When this had happened a few times in the past, it indicated there might be a silent, deadly buildup of iron in my liver from one of the medical conditions I had called "Hemochromatosis[1]". This condition causes the body to store too much iron.

Clinical tests I had years earlier confirmed I had active Hemochromatosis requiring that I had to donate a pint of blood every eight weeks to reduce the level of iron in my body. If I did not have the required phlebotomies, this condition would lead to an overload of iron in my liver and other organs, and would ultimately destroy the liver and lead to certain death.

At this consult, Dr. Hertz was especially concerned when I told him how I had been feeling increasingly ill and lethargic over the prior recent weeks ... and had unintentionally lost more than ten pounds in two weeks. Dr. Hertz ordered a special scan of my abdomen, a MRI-MRCP[2] with "T-cell equipment." This was to scan my entire abdomen (with and without contrast) to determine if there was a buildup of iron in my liver as happened years earlier. The doctor also drew blood to run a number of other tests.

The MRI-MRCP was done at Zwanger-Pesiri Radiology in Massapequa, Long Island. Interestingly, the scan was scheduled to

---

[1] **Hemochromatosis** – This is a condition where a gene called HFE is most often the cause of hereditary hemochromatosis. You inherit one HFE gene from each of your parents. The HFE gene has two common mutations, C282Y and H63D. Genetic testing can reveal whether you have these mutations in your HFE gene.

[2] **MRCP** - Magnetic Resonance Cholangiopancreatography is a non-invasive MRI exam used to visualize the bile ducts, pancreatic duct and the pancreas.

be done at three o'clock, the hour of "Divine Mercy."

For those who may not be familiar with Divine Mercy, it is a Catholic devotion to Jesus Christ initiated by the apparitions of Jesus as revealed to Saint Faustina Kowalska. This devotion is recognized, in part, by the highly venerated image of Christ with rays streaming out from His heart representing the unlimited, merciful love of God toward all people. The three main themes of the Divine Mercy devotion include:
- To ask for and obtain the mercy of God;
- To trust in Christ's abundant mercy, and finally,
- To show mercy to others and act as a conduit for God's mercy toward them.

A few days later, the radiology report of my MRI-MRCP scan had some surprising, terrible news. The good news was that there was NO sign of iron-buildup in my liver. The bad news was that there was strong evidence I had something terribly wrong in my biliary tree and common bile duct near my pancreas. This news did not sound very good; I was taken completely by surprise. I wondered what could possibly be causing this?

The next time I saw Dr. Hertz, he read the radiology report from Zwanger-Pesiri that ominously stated there were a number of areas in my abdomen that required further tests to rule out what was called, "periampullary lesion of the biliary tree and pancreas."

"Oh, my God," I thought, "not another cancer!"

The look on Dr. Hertz's face did not help me feel any better. He was clearly quite concerned as he recommended that I immediately follow-up right away. He recommended I make an appointment for a consultation with Dr. Rajiv Bansal, a highly regarded gastroenterologist, at North Shore Hospital in Lake Success, Long Island, New York.

A few days later on February 17, 2017, my wife, Margie, and I were sitting in Dr. Rajiv Bansal's office as he showed us MRI images of my abdomen on a special MRI reader in his office. After stressing how badly my entire biliary system was distended, he pointed to an area that was clearly blocking my entire biliary system.

He explained, "Whatever that blockage is, it is quite serious. It has your entire biliary system badly distended ... and has caused your gallbladder, liver and pancreas to swell up dangerously! The blockage appears to be situated right at the location of your ampulla of vater at the bottom of your common bile duct outside your pancreas."

Dr. Bansal also noted that a CD I had given him of a CT/PET scan of my abdomen done at the Columbia Hospital Cancer Center in late 2009 showed there were six (6) growths in my gallbladder at that time! Dr. Bansal said this was very confusing because none of those six growths showed up as still being there on the recent February 10, 2017 MRI-MRCP scan.

"I don't think those growths were tumors since they are no longer seen on your recent MRI. They might have been gallstones which passed since 2009. Having said that, given their size, they likely would have greatly irritated your biliary tree ... and I do not see how they could possibly have passed through your ampulla of vater. If they did, they would have badly scraped your ampulla and caused great scarring as they passed through. This is all quite mysterious."

After saying this, Dr. Bansal dramatically shook his head and stated, "Yeah that could not have happened. Those six gallstones on the 2009 CT/PET scan were way too large to pass! There is no way they could have passed through your system. That's not even remotely possible."

MY JOURNEY WITH NEUROENDOCRINE CANCER
What You Don't Know Can Kill You!

After a pause, he muttered, "But then ... what happened to them? Where did they go?"

I told him, "The only reasonable explanation is what I and family members believe. We believe God removed those growths in my gallbladder in response to many prayers and Masses that were offered for me at that time."

The doctor smiled and simply said he was going to schedule an endoscopy with EUS[3] and ERCP[4] to allow him to "see what exactly is going on in your abdomen ... and ... to rule out the possibility of periampullary cancer."

Prior to having this procedure, Margie and I joined other family members on February 20, 2017 for a two-day trip to Washington D.C. to visit one of our grandsons, Bobby Walsh. On the second day of the trip, I awoke feeling outrageously ill with a headache, nausea, chills, weakness and lethargy. I was so sick, my older son, Rob, did all the driving on our way home to Long Island. The emotional strain of not knowing what was happening to me added yet another frightening dimension to my suffering.

Feeling desperately ill, and having already survived two other unrelated, malignant cancers, I wondered if one of those earlier cancers had now returned ... or worse yet ... was this another, new type of cancer?

This, "we don't know yet stage," is another part of the heavy cross we cancer patients often carry on our painful journey.

---

[3] **EUS** – **E**ndoscopic **U**ltra**s**ound combines endoscopy and ultrasound to obtain images and information about the digestive tract and the surrounding tissue and organs.

[4] **ERCP** - **E**ndoscopic **R**etrograde **C**holangio **P**ancreatography is a procedure used to diagnose diseases of the gallbladder, biliary system, pancreas and liver. The test actually looks upward where digestive fluids come from (the liver, gallbladder and pancreas) and down to where the fluids enter the intestines.

BOB WALSH

Chapter 2

"THERE'S BLEEDING INSIDE YOUR EYE"

A few days before Dr. Raj Bansal was to do a special endoscope procedure to learn what was causing the terrible, excruciating pain in my abdomen, I woke up, opened my eyes and was startled to discover I had a new, very serious, unrelated health crisis. The sight in my right eye was almost completely blocked by a large, gray area in the very center of my field of vision!

"What now?" I worried. "Is this trouble with my eyesight related to what is going on in my abdomen? What in God's name is happening to me?"

After composing myself, I was relieved that the vision in my left eye was okay ... at least at the time.

"Well, if I'm going to lose the sight in my right eye, at least my left eye still works," I comforted myself. "Besides, whatever is wrong with my right eye may only be temporary."

Rather than worry, I focused instead on what St. Padre Pio[5] once said how we can view times of personal suffering. He said, "If you could see all the good that comes from offering your sufferings up for the benefit of the holy souls in Purgatory, you might not ask God to take away those sufferings!"

With St. Pio's words in mind, I offered up my fears and sufferings for the benefit of the holy souls in Purgatory ... and made an emergency appointment that day with Dr. Gregory Persak. Dr. Persak is a highly regarded ophthalmologist at the Center for Eye

---

[5] **St. Padre Pio** – He was an Italian priest in the Catholic faith with an extraordinary healing gift. For fifty years, he had the gift of the stigmata - the five wounds of Christ. He was born Francesco Forgione on May 25, 1887 in Pietrelcina, Italy, and died on September 23, 1968.

Care in West Islip, Long Island, New York. After running several diagnostic tests, the doctor delivered some disturbing news.

"It appears you have 'wet macular degeneration[6]' of your right eye."

Dr. Persak explained, "Your left eye appears to be okay ... at least for now. The condition in your right eye, however, is quite serious, Mr. Walsh. You need to have it treated right away by one of our specialists."

I immediately made the necessary appointment ... and added this new health crisis to my prayers at daily Mass.

Two days later, I went see (no pun intended) Dr. Matthew Strachovsky, an ophthalmologist and retina specialist at the same Center for Eye Care in West Islip. After conducting a number of specialized tests, the doctor confirmed that I did, indeed, have "wet macular degeneration" in my right eye.

The doctor explained, "Unfortunately, you have abnormal capillaries in your right eye which are bleeding into the interior of your eye. I recommend you immediately begin having a series of three monthly injections of an anti-coagulant called 'Avastin' in your right eye in an attempt to close the abnormal bleeding capillaries."

He said the injections of Avastin might stop and/or slow down the bleeding that was happening inside my right eye.

"There is no assurance the Avastin will work to close up the tiny, abnormal capillaries that are bleeding. The bleeding, in turn, unfortunately causes scarring. Avastin might help to stop the bleeding and thereby avoid further scarring ... and further loss of vision in that eye."

---

[6] **Wet Macular Degeneration** - This is a progressive eye condition that damages the macula, the part of the retina that is responsible for central vision. As abnormal blood vessels bleed, the blood builds up and can cause visual distortions that can lead to the loss of central vision.

MY JOURNEY WITH NEUROENDOCRINE CANCER
What You Don't Know Can Kill You!

Dr. Strachovsky added that, over time, the body should slowly, gradually, absorb the blood that had already accumulated inside my eye. The doctor further explained how the injections into my eye would be done. He first injects the eye with a mild anesthetic so I would only feel a little pressure in the eye when he injects the eye with Avastin.

To agree to have a monthly needle directly injected into my eye was not a welcome thought, but under the dire circumstances I found myself in, it was an easy decision to proceed. After all, I really did not have much choice. Either I agreed to get injections in my right eye and hope it worked to save my eyesight, or, the sight in that eye would be permanently lost. I agreed and immediately scheduled to begin the monthly injections in my eye.

Rather than allowing this additional, depressing news to pull us down, my wife, Margie, and I responded with additional prayer and daily Mass. These days were our time to "walk on the water" like St. Peter did when Jesus called him to walk on the water during a storm at sea. In the midst of the frightening storm raging around us - worrying about yet another malignant cancer and loss of the sight in my right eye ... among other things – Margie and I chose to keep our eyes firmly set on Jesus.

I reassured Margie, "I might lose my physical sight, but as long as I have my spiritual sight, we will be just fine!"

"I fully agree, Bob," Margie in turn reassured me.

Thank God we did ... the storm enveloping us was about to get much, much worse.

BOB WALSH

Chapter 3

"A TUMOR IS BLOCKING EVERYTHING!"

On February 27, 2017, just a few days after learning I was likely going to lose the sight in my right eye, I found myself lying on a hard, ice cold table in an operating room at North Shore Hospital in Manhasset, Long Island, New York. I was there to find out if there was a malignant cancer blocking my entire biliary system.

To determine this, Dr. Rajiv Bansal was about to perform a special endoscopy procedure with what they call "EUS" and "ERCP." This procedure is a highly effective method that allows doctors to see inside the digestive system without having to cut into the body from outside the torso. The primary goal of this procedure was to allow Dr. Bansal to determine what was causing the blockage in my abdomen. Going in, the doctor already knew from the MRI done two weeks prior that there was a virtual, complete blockage of my entire biliary system causing a grotesque distension of my biliary tracts, my gallbladder, liver and pancreas.

Like so many cancer patients who go through various operations and surgical procedures, I felt so vulnerable and wondered what, if anything, the doctor was going to discover. And what, if anything, will the doctor have to surgically remove while I was unconscious?

"When I wake up," I wondered, "will I be in the recovery room ... or will I be standing in front of Almighty God?" Due to several other serious conditions I have, there was a chance I might not wake up from the procedure.

These last-second thoughts raced through my mind as I was about to be put out under general anesthesia. I asked God to forgive me all the sins of my life, and have mercy on me if this was the time my physical life would end. I also asked God to please look after all my loved ones for me. After praying these thoughts, a powerful sense of peace and confidence descended upon me.

I asked Dr. Bansal and the other operating room attendants to please wait a moment so I could pray for them and for all the other people who have serious health issues. To my surprise and delight, Dr. Bansal and the others in the operating room stopped what they were doing and stood around me as I prayed! What a wonderful, reassuring experience as the anesthesia then swirled in and took effect.

Later, when I awoke in the recovery room, my wife, Margie, and my daughter, Peggie, were by my side. We eagerly waited for Dr. Bansal to come tell us what he discovered during the procedure. I fully expected it was not likely going to be good news … but I was comforted with the thought that I was finally going to find out what was wrong and what was causing so much pain and suffering.

When Dr. Bansal arrived, he immediately shared what he discovered.

"A tumor is blocking everything!" he dramatically stated. "When I got to your ampulla of vater, I saw it was completely closed so I had to cut it in order to open everything up. Once I did, all the bile that had been backed up by the blockage flowed down quite freely."

My immediate reaction was relief. "That's good news, doctor; that's very good news. That explains why I have had such terrible pain in my abdomen. Everything was backed up and distended from the blockage at my ampulla."

A concerned look on Dr. Bansal's face told me there was more to this story. Looking downward, he clearly was struggling to find the right words to say. An uncomfortable silence followed as Margie, Peggie and I each noticed the unmistakable worried look on the doctor's face.

MY JOURNEY WITH NEUROENDOCRINE CANCER
What You Don't Know Can Kill You!

Margie broke the ice by bluntly asking, "What is it, doctor? What's wrong?"

When Dr. Bansal did not answer, Margie insisted, "Look, doctor, something is obviously bothering you. What did you find?"

"Oh boy," I thought, "here it comes! Something pretty bad must be coming. I wonder if that blockage was another type of cancer?"

Carefully choosing his words, Dr. Bansal spoke softly, "Once I opened your ampulla of vater, Mr. Walsh, I saw a tumor on the other side. That is what was blocking your entire biliary system and why your organs were so swollen."

Before letting this alarming news to fully set in, he quickly blurted out, "It was a benign tumor. Although it was quite small, the tumor nevertheless was able to block up everything."

Before I, Margie or Peggie could ask any questions, he added, "I took several pictures and biopsies of the tumor and the entire surrounding area. When the pathology report on the biopsies comes in, I will give you a call and let you know exactly what the pathologists have to say."

Before we could ask any questions, Dr. Bansal turned and quickly left the area giving us the impression he did not want to answer any questions. Margie, Peggie and I were stunned but relieved to hear Dr. Bansal tell us the tumor was benign.

I wondered if what the doctor saw in me was really only benign. Was it possible the tumor was malignant, I worried. Given the significant level of pain and suffering I endure, I could not help but think this might well be the beginning of the end for me. Like other cancer patients who find themselves in such a terrible position, this "waiting and not knowing" is one of the torturous stages of cancer for us and our families.

Although I did not yet know if the tumor was malignant, deep down inside, I sensed my life as I knew it was never going to be the same again. Rather than living in fear and despair, however, I continued to live in faith and hope, pray and attend Masses, and offer my sufferings for the benefit of holy souls in Purgatory.

Chapter 4

"THERE'S MORE BLEEDING IN YOUR EYE!"

Every day was like an eternity as I and my family anxiously waited for Dr. Bansal to call with results of the biopsies of the tumor he found blocking my entire biliary system. In the meantime, I had an appointment with Dr. Strachovsky, my ophthalmologist. At this visit, the doctor planned to inject my right eye with a needle filled with Avastin medicine in the hopes the Avastin would stop - or slow down - the progression of the wet macular degeneration bleeding in my right eye.

At his office, several diagnostic tests were first conducted to determine how the wet macular degeneration was progressing. The results of these tests would more clearly indicate to him whether or not I was likely going to lose all the sight in my right eye - with or without Avastin injections.

All my recent, serious health issues had me feeling so vulnerable and defenseless. It seemed like only yesterday that I was enjoying the relatively simple ways of life. Now, I found myself to be one of those unfortunate people forced to sit on pins and needles waiting to hear whether or not I had malignant cancer ... and whether or not I was also going to lose the sight in my right eye.

"Waiting to hear," I was painfully learning, was yet another utterly torturous stage that often accompanies serious health issues. However, being a life-long, faith-filled Catholic, my reaction to all this was to turn ever more so to God through prayer and daily Mass. I simply was not going to give in to worry and despair; I chose instead - Confession, Mass and Holy Communion.

When Dr. Strachovsky entered the room, he clearly appeared very concerned about something as he sat down to give me the results of the latest tests he ran on both my eyes.

"I am afraid the wet macular degeneration in your right eye has become even worse than before, Mr. Walsh. There's a lot more new bleeding in that eye!"

As if that news was not bad enough, he added, "I am so sorry to tell you the scarring in the eye is **ALSO** ... much worse!"

"What is the significance of all that?" I asked.

He looked surprised by my question.

"As I explained last time, Mr. Walsh, it indicates that you are likely going to lose more and more of the sight in that eye as the bleeding continues. The loss of sight is a direct result of scarring that is caused by the bleeding, and that, I hope you remember, Mr. Walsh ... is **NOT** reversible."

"Okay," I thought. "I do trust you, God, but all this is getting very, very scary!"

Realizing there was nothing I could do about all the crazy things happening to me with the cancer and loss of eyesight, I decided to do what **I COULD DO** ... I continued to turn to God and renewed my prayers for His help. I made sure to ask everyone I knew – family, friends and rosarians in Ss. Cyril and Methodius and St. Matthew's parishes – to join my prayers.

"Dear God, I know there's not much **I** can do about all the crazy things happening to me ... but I know **YOU CAN**! I trust you, Lord, and I know you are able to heal me, and so, that is what I ask. If that is not Your will at this time, Lord, please fill me with the graces needed to be strong and courageous through it all. Whatever comes, comes! I know I am going to be okay because You said You are with us at all times."

After Dr. Strachovsky explained once again how he first uses a needle filled with anesthetic medicine, he then used it to inject the medicine directly into the lower right corner of my right eye. I was so nervous about having a needle stuck in my eye but I reminded myself that this was the only hope I had to save the sight

MY JOURNEY WITH NEUROENDOCRINE CANCER
What You Don't Know Can Kill You!

in my eye. I really had no choice.

I put everything out of my mind except prayer ... and stayed as still as I could. I was pleasantly surprised that I barely felt the needle go into my eye. Dr. Strachovsky waited a few minutes for the anesthesia to fully set in, then he slowly approached me from the right as he instructed me to keep my eye wide open ... and remain as still as possible.

I prayed to God for mercy and strength to deal with what I expected was going to be terrible pain. Staying as perfectly still as I could, I even held my breath as Dr. Strachovsky stuck the needle into the far lower right corner of my open right eye. As he did, the needle released the anti-coagulant medicine, Avastin, into my eye.

I barely felt anything!

"Oh, thank you, God," I silently prayed as I felt like an enormous weight had been lifted off me.

Despite this feeling of relief, I wondered, "Is all this going to work? Is it worth getting needles stuck in my eye? Are the injections going to save my sight ... or am I going to lose my sight anyway?"

I still had to worry that I was going to need some painful, excruciating surgery if my "benign" biopsies are, in fact, malignant. As those frightening, depressing thoughts cascaded together, I strongly suspected it all might be coming from the Devil in its attempts to drive me to despair ... and away from God.

I knew if I was going to survive and enjoy any quality of life, I had to resist self-pitying thoughts, and stay focused on Jesus - no matter what may come my way. Those days were certainly some of the toughest, most challenging times of my life as one heavy cross after another piled on testing the strength of my faith and that of my family and friends. I resolved once again that I was going to continue to walk on the water like St. Peter did ... and keep my eyes steadfastly on Jesus.

BOB WALSH

Thank God I did … things were about to get even worse.

Chapter 5

BECOMING A "ZEBRA"

On March 9, 2017, a few days after I received the first needle of Avastin injected into my right eye, my gastroenterologist, Dr. Rajiv Bansal, called to tell me pathology results of the biopsies he removed from my biliary system weeks earlier.

The doctor reported, "The biopsies show it was benign!"

These words brought great relief for me, family and friends ... but not for long.

I later learned to my great surprise that Dr. Bansal was totally mistaken! The North Shore Hospital's surgical pathology report dated March 1, 2017, in fact, clearly stated that the tumor biopsied was "a well-differentiated neuroendocrine neoplasm located on the ampulla of vater!"

To this day, I do not understand how Dr. Bansal twice mistakenly told me the tumor was benign! He initially said this in the recovery room at North Shore Hospital immediately following the endoscopy on February 27, 2017. The second time was on March 9, 2017 when he called saying he received the pathology results indicating the tumor was benign.

When I later confronted him with his inexplicable, serious misstatements, he stunned me by saying matter-of-factly, "Well ... most tumors like the one you have usually turn out to be benign!"

I told him this was terribly unprofessional and asked why he did not wait to get the official pathology report rather than taking it upon himself to make such an inappropriate assumption over something so very important. He did not answer ... nor did he offer an apology. Unbelievable!

The pathology report by the way was signed by two different North Shore Hospital pathologists confirming that I did, indeed, have a rare, malignant neuroendocrine tumor (NET) located in my common bile duct by my ampulla of vater ... immediately adjacent to my pancreas.

The pathologists also noted there was a growth in the antrum (lower-most part) of my stomach which they ominously stated was a "pre-cancerous lesion." The report went on to state that the rest of my digestive system was in serious condition since the NET tumor had virtually closed off the common bile duct. This resulted in several potentially fatal conditions:

- There was a serious backup of ever-expanding digestive fluids from the gallbladder, liver and pancreas. All the bile fluids were blocked off by the NET tumor located on my ampulla of vater;
- There was a serious distension of the gallbladder; and,
- There was a grotesque distension of the entire biliary tree caused by the blockage of the ampulla of vater by the NET tumor.

Subsequently, in a conversation with a NET cancer patient, she said, "Congratulations, Bob, you are now a fellow zebra!"

"What do you mean? Why are you saying I am now a zebra?" I asked.

She explained, "People with neuroendocrine cancer are called zebras. The reason a zebra is a symbol for people like us who have neuroendocrine cancer is because doctors usually misdiagnose symptoms as coming from other conditions ... rather than NET cancer. It is like when someone hears hoof-beats. Nine of ten people think the sounds are from horses - rather than from other sources that make hoof-beat sounds ... like zebras!

"Actually, the term, 'zebra,' is universally accepted as a reference to any rare disease or condition. You know, like neuroendocrine cancer!"

MY JOURNEY WITH NEUROENDOCRINE CANCER
What You Don't Know Can Kill You!

This fellow zebra ominously warned me, "It is inevitable that you - like other NET cancer patients - are going to have some doctor misinterpret your symptoms, misstate critical information … and possibly even mistreat you."

BOB WALSH

MY JOURNEY WITH NEUROENDOCRINE CANCER
What You Don't Know Can Kill You!

Chapter 6

"YOU NEED THE WHIPPLE!"

Soon after reading the pathology report from North Shore Hospital pathologists confirming I had neuroendocrine cancer, I made an appointment for a second opinion with Dr. Dmitri Alden, a surgical oncologist reportedly familiar with the treatment of neuroendocrine cancer.

In preparation for this consult set for March 20, 2017, I arranged ahead of time to personally pick up the biopsy slides of my NET cancer. After signing a number of forms to take possession of my biopsy slides at Dr. Bansal's office, I drove from his Lake Success office on Long Island to Dr. Alden's office at 186 East 76th Street in Manhattan. In addition to my biopsy slides, I dropped off all my related MRI CDs, pathology and radiology reports, related medical reports and a large number of papers I completed the night before.

One of the most annoying, frustrating things we cancer patients endure is the seemingly endless ordeal of filling out countless forms and documents at doctors' offices! That is a close second, of course, to making an appointment with a doctor ... or should I say ... trying to make an appointment.

Using the telephone these days, you often have to listen to unwanted, annoying information before you finally get to speak to a human being who can actually help with the simple reason you are calling. If you do not already have hypertension, by the time you finally accomplish the simple reason for your call, you will probably need blood pressure medication!

With an appointment for a second opinion in hand, I hoped to hear some encouraging news about what I might be able to do to battle the deadly cancer I had growing inside me. Like most patients dealing with incurable, malignant cancer, I was ready and eager to grab onto anything positive or encouraging ... anything.

"Perhaps we will hear something encouraging today about what we can do," my wife, Margie, optimistically said.

How wrong she was.

We travelled to New York City by car for the consultation with Dr. Dmitri Alden. On our way in, we took turns speaking optimistically about how it was, in fact, entirely possible that we might hear something encouraging about what could be done to deal with the rare, incurable neuroendocrine cancer. As usual when we drive anywhere, we also made time to pray the Rosary.

By the time we reached the city and parked in a garage close to Dr. Alden's office, we were feeling upbeat. After waiting a short time, we were escorted into the doctor's office. I was immediately impressed with the doctor's relaxed, gentle appearance and manner.

After politely greeting us, Dr. Alden began calmly stating he thoroughly reviewed all my records including that of Lenox Hill Hospital's highly skilled pathologists. He stressed how carefully they analyzed my biopsy slides.

Easing comfortably back into his chair, Dr. Alden looked me right in the eyes and said, "Mr. Walsh, you unfortunately have neuroendocrine cancer ... a most rare and incurable cancer!"

I immediately began to realize this was NOT going to the hope-filled visit Margie and I had hoped it would be.

Without hesitation, Dr. Alden added, "You probably have had this cancer for many years and now it has reached a serious, potentially lethal stage."

The doctor paused to allow Margie and me to ask questions. I immediately bombarded him with one question after another.

"Doctor, I've never heard of neuroendocrine cancer. If this is as rare as you say, how can you be so sure I have it? What kind of cancer is it anyway? How do I treat it? How about chemo? Why don't you just cut it out?"

The doctor smiled and went about clearly answering each question - one at a time. The bottom line he stressed was there was no doubt about me having neuroendocrine cancer.

Like so many people who receive such terrible, devastating news, my next thought was, "I wonder if this neuroendocrine cancer is the reason why I have suffered so badly in mysterious ways throughout my life?"

The many doctors and specialists I conferred with over the years were never able to diagnose what was causing several painful symptoms I suffered with - especially those involving my digestive system. I suffered cramps, bloating, gas, along with a steady, debilitating, painful leakage of blood and caustic, acid-like fluid from my rectum. The leaking fluids severely burned my rectum and the surrounding area. The more I walked, the more heavily the leakage poured out.

In addition, there were two other health issues no doctor could ever diagnose. One was the excruciating pain I felt in the thoracic area of my back (the middle center area) whenever I would lie down on a hard, flat surface. MRIs, CT scans and X-rays all failed to indicate the source of the agonizing pain. (I also have a NET lesion on my spine!)

The second mystery centered around the fact that virtually every blood test I had during the prior 20 years showed I had a very low red blood count, and extremely low vitamin D level.

Dr. Alden stated it was neuroendocrine cancer that was at the root cause of painful rectal leakage, debilitating thoracic back pain (from the NET lesion), low red blood count, low vitamin D level and other issues.

I told Dr. Alden how for many years, my former primary care physician, Dr. Marc Lewandoski, in Deer Park, New York, ran comprehensive blood tests that consistently showed seriously low red blood count and vitamin D levels. "Dr. Lewandoski never pursued the underlying reason for this. Instead, he always assured me that some people simply have very low level red blood count and Vitamin D!"

Dr. Alden shook his head and scoffed, "That's terrible. The doctors treating you over the years should have questioned such low levels as possible signs of neuroendocrine cancer. That is so unfortunate. With malignant cancer, timing is so important. The sooner it is discovered and treatments begin, the greater your chances of surviving it."

"Great," I thought, "So how late is it, doctor? What can I do now?" I asked.

Without hesitation, he firmly stated, "Mr. Walsh, you need 'Whipple' surgery."

Margie and I were there only a few minutes and already I was terribly distraught.

Dr. Alden thoroughly explained why he thought I needed the Whipple surgical procedure. Pausing for only a moment to allow the disturbing news to set in, the doctor proceeded to describe what this surgical procedure entails.

"The cancerous area including the ampulla of vater must be removed along with part of your common bile duct, your gallbladder, about 40% of your pancreas, part of the duodenum and lymph nodes! What remains in the area must then be surgically reconstructed!"

"This is scary and terribly depressing, doctor!" I complained. "There has to be something else I can do."

Just when I thought what the doctor was saying could not possibly get much worse, Dr. Alden ominously added, "You know, Mr. Walsh, given your age and other health conditions, there's no guarantee a patient like you would survive such traumatic surgery!"

MY JOURNEY WITH NEUROENDOCRINE CANCER
What You Don't Know Can Kill You!

Without having to be asked, he enumerated a number of reasons for such a dire outlook.

"The first reason has to do with where the NET tumor is located in your body; it's right on the ampulla of vater. Look at how it closed up your entire biliary system. That alone is quite serious. A second reason is that you have many other serious health conditions. Any one of them could cause very serious complications. What's more, you have extensive scar tissue from all the prior surgeries you have had.

"By the way, to work around your hernia-mesh and scar tissues, for the Whipple surgery I would have to enter your torso by making a horizontal incision across the upper part of your torso ... rather than making the conventional vertical incision to access the area. The entire Whipple procedure - without complications - would require several hours to complete. Those are just some of the **MAJOR** factors involved, Mr. Walsh. There are other ... less serious ... though important factors to be considered."

Almost as an afterthought, Dr. Alden added, "In case you are wondering, doing the Whipple surgery might only add a few years to your life. If I were to guess, I would say five years at most."

"Five? Only five? You guess?" I complained.

Looking directly at me, he bluntly stated, "Yes, Mr. Walsh ... five years ... and very likely less than that. You have to remember, what you have is a deadly, incurable malignancy. And although it's a very slow-growing cancer, you probably have had it most of your adult life. It has now reached a critical stage."

Margie and I could not believe what we were hearing!

Dr. Alden cautioned, "The longer you wait to have the Whipple surgery, the more difficult the surgery will be ... and the less likely you will survive the operation!"

After Dr. Alden answered our questions, he handed me a number of prescriptions to have special blood and urine tests done, and a "Gallium-68" CT/PET scan. He said these tests should be done as soon as possible ... whether or not I decided to have the Whipple surgery. We thanked Dr. Alden and agreed to call him in a day or two with our decision on whether or not I would have the Whipple surgery.

Margie, and I left Dr. Alden's office feeling far more depressed and worried than when we arrived. Neither of us spoke a word as we slowly walked along 76th Street on our way to the nearby parking garage. We had gone only a short distance when my guardian angel reminded me that we were literally just around the corner from Saint Anne's Shrine in St. Jean the Baptiste Church on Lexington Avenue and 76th Street.

I stopped walking and told Margie, "Saint Anne's Shrine is just around the corner. After what we just heard, we **HAVE** to go for a visit."

"But, it will be rush-hour soon, Bob. If we don't leave right now, the traffic will be horrendous," she lamented.

"I know, Margie, but Jesus should be there on exposition in the monstrance on the main altar ... and we just got such terrible news from Dr. Alden. We have to make time to visit God ... and to ask Him to help us!"

Margie didn't need any more convincing as we turned and quickly walked the short distance to St. Jean the Baptiste Church. Thank God we did ... something quite miraculous was about to happen there.

Chapter 7

MIRACLE AT SAINT ANNE'S SHRINE IN NEW YORK CITY

It was three o'clock, the hour of Divine Mercy, as Margie and I slowly climbed up the front steps of St. Jean the Baptiste Church on Lexington Avenue and 76th Street in Manhattan. Our hearts were heavy from devastating news we had just received from the oncologist, Dr. Alden, who recommended I have the extensive surgery known as the "Whipple" procedure.

St. Jean the Baptiste Church is located in the heart of midtown New York City. It is famous throughout the Catholic world, in part, because a relic of Saint Anne, grandmother of Jesus Christ, is maintained there. The relic is from Saint Anne's forearm which Catholic tradition states once held the baby Jesus. The relic is maintained in a glass reliquary immediately adjacent to a shrine dedicated to Saint Anne and the Blessed Mother.

Since I grew up in this area of New York City, I and my family were quite familiar with this church and Saint Anne's Shrine. In fact, for many years I had taken scores of people to the Shrine for healing prayer ... and witnessed countless miraculous healings.

As I entered the magnificent church this time, however, there was a distinct difference from prior visits over the years. This time, I was the one who desperately needed healing. The new feeling faded when I could see that Jesus was present in the Eucharist in a monstrance on the main altar all the way up front in the church. To my great surprise, Margie stood perfectly still in the center aisle as she began complaining to Jesus.

"Are you kidding me?" she snapped. **"You didn't answer my prayers!** Now Bob has to have some life-threatening surgery!"

While Margie was having her "discussion" with Jesus, I decided to walk quietly over to the beautiful, pure-white marble, life-size statue of Saint Anne and the Blessed Mother located in an alcove in the right rear (southwest) corner of the church. Standing there, my mind was filled with frightening thoughts of the terrible situation I so suddenly found myself in. I felt so helpless as I confessed how worried I was about the deadly NET cancer growing inside me … and what it was likely going to do to me.

I realized the neuroendocrine cancer had deeply entrenched itself inside me like a living, violent creature feeding on me. It had nearly killed me already. Will I have to go through torturous surgeries? Are doctors going to have to cut me up just to give me a little more time to live? If so, how long? Is this NET cancer really going to kill me? My poor wife and family are going to suffer watching what this cancer will do to me.

NET cancer is one gigantic, cruel bully … and it seems there is nothing I could do about it. Such upsetting thoughts left me feeling so very, very depressed. I realized how other NET cancer patients must be tortured with similar thoughts and worries. How many, I wondered, turn to God when the sufferings caused by NET cancer overwhelm them – perhaps especially that feeling of helplessness.

These thoughts led me to think of how Jesus suffered in the Garden of Gethsemane. I envisioned Him kneeling there … feeling alone in those moments of terrible, indescribable suffering.

Knowing He would understand what I was going through, I called out to Him from the inner recesses of my heart, "Dear Jesus, You asked God the Father if the cup of suffering might pass from You without having to drink from it. I follow your example, Jesus, by now asking God the Father - through You - to please let this cup of suffering pass from me.

MY JOURNEY WITH NEUROENDOCRINE CANCER
What You Don't Know Can Kill You!

"If I must suffer from this cancer, please let it be that I will not require the Whipple surgery. Perhaps, I can only have some chemo."

After a pause, I reluctantly added, "But as You said, Jesus, I, too, say, 'Your will be done, Father, not mine.' If I am not to be healed of this cancer, then please bless me with the graces I am going to need to endure the agony I see coming my way. In a like way, I pray for all the other people who are suffering from the ravages of cancer."

As I stood there, I recalled some of the many times over the years I stood in that very same spot in front of the statue with people who were suffering with some terrible illness. The first one that came to mind was a middle-aged man by the name of Hector who had forty tumors throughout his heart and lungs. Sloan Kettering Memorial Hospital had given him only a few months to live when he asked me to pray over him asking God to heal him.

After attending Mass, Hector and I stood in front of Saint Anne's Shrine where I asked her and the Blessed Mother to intercede with Jesus for Hector's healing. As we prayed, the statue of Saint Anne and the Blessed Mother began to turn a vibrant pink color! At that very moment, an exhilarating tingling sensation swept over Hector and me.

The following week a whole body CT/PET scan at Sloan Kettering showed that all of the tumors in Hector's heart and lungs were gone; all that remained were tiny pin dots where each of the tumors had been! Remembering this - and other similar, remarkable miracles – I turned to my beloved patron saint, Saint Anne, and her daughter, the Blessed Mother Mary, and asked them to intercede on my behalf with Jesus.

"I know how much Jesus loves you. Please ask Him to hear my prayers and have mercy on me."

At that moment, my guardian angel surprised me by encouraging me to use my cell phone to take a photo of the statue of Saint Anne and the Blessed Mother. After I took the picture, my guardian angel surprised me once again by urging me to take yet another picture of the statue! I did so without hesitation because I have learned over the years to do what my angel suggests or encourages me to do. When I looked at the two pictures, I was amazed to see that a remarkable miracle was captured.

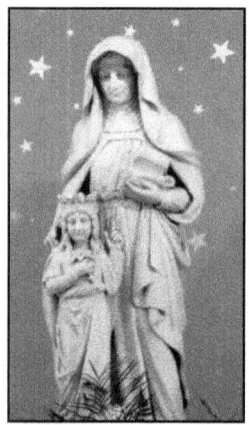

In the first photo shown on the left, Saint Anne's head on the statue can clearly be seen looking downward off to her right side. Also, the eyes of the Blessed Mother can be seen looking downward. This is how the statue has been - unchanged - for well over 100 years since it was created in Italy and transported by transatlantic cargo ship to St. Jean the Baptiste Church on 76th Street and Lexington Avenue in New York City.

In the second photo shown on the right, I was surprised to see that the statue of Saint Anne and the Blessed Mother were then looking directly at me! I was absolutely mesmerized. Then I noticed there appeared to be many more stars now on the wall behind the statue. As I studied them, I recalled the Catholic tradition that tells us Saint Anne was among those who travelled to Bethlehem when Jesus was born. Part of that tradition also believes

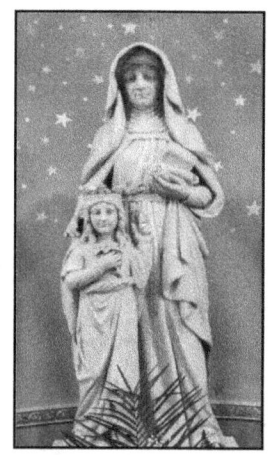

Saint Anne was one of the first to cradle the Christ Child in her arms.

MY JOURNEY WITH NEUROENDOCRINE CANCER
What You Don't Know Can Kill You!

Basking in that glorious moment, my worries and concerns about having neuroendocrine cancer and the dreaded Whipple surgery were replaced with feelings of peace and security.

As captured in the two remarkable photos, it was clear that Saint Anne and the Blessed Mother wanted to make sure I knew they heard my cries for help. This extraordinary miracle lifted my spirits for the painful, difficult times ahead.

How I wish everyone who carries the cross of cancer could be so blessed.

BOB WALSH

MY JOURNEY WITH NEUROENDOCRINE CANCER
What You Don't Know Can Kill You!

Chapter 8

"I HAVE OTHER PATIENTS WITH REAL CANCER!"

The above shocking words were actually said to me and my wife, Margie, by an oncologist, Dr. John Allendorf, at a consultation in his Mineola, New York office in March 2017. I can only assume his words were meant to ease our fears and concerns over having neuroendocrine cancer.

I made this appointment because Dr. Allendorf was considered by many as one of the best pancreatic cancer specialists on Long Island where I lived. However, like other oncologists at the time, the doctor's words showed how little he regarded neuroendocrine cancer compared other types of malignant cancers. He said NET cancer was the slowest growing of all, and its tumors rarely become very large.

His opinion ignored the fact that weeks earlier, one of these "slow growing, small NET tumors" nearly ended my life.

Unfortunately for me and other neuroendocrine cancer patients, this experience is not uncommon. We have found that many oncologists have similar opinions when it comes to neuroendocrine cancer. This highlights one of the greatest challenges for us NET cancer patients - that is to find an oncologist with understanding of - experience dealing with - neuroendocrine cancer.

For us, this can be the difference between life and death.

As my journey with NET cancer progressed, I heard from other NET cancer patients how misinformation on the part of their doctors was quite common. Fellow cancer patients scoffed at what I experienced, saying they had endured far worse at the hands of their oncologists.

When I called to make an appointment with Dr. Allendorf, I

asked if the doctor was familiar with neuroendocrine cancer.

The reply was, "Yes, he is ... how do you spell that cancer?"

After I spelled it, I was assured the doctor was among the very best oncologists and was certainly familiar with the ... "type of cancer you have."

Friends in the NET cancer community later advised me that the type of phone exchange should have alerted me to make further inquiries to determine if the oncologist was really familiar with neuroendocrine cancer.

"If the person scheduling appointments for the oncologist apparently hasn't heard of neuroendocrine cancer, then chances are the oncologist hasn't either!" Unfortunately for me, I was so desperate at the time to find an oncologist, ANY oncologist, who could provide additional advice on how to deal with the NET cancer, I went ahead and made the appointment.

My encounter with Dr. Allendorf began only a few days after Margie and I had visited Dr. Alden and Saint Anne's Shrine in New York City. During our drive to see Dr. Allendorf, we prayed the Rosary and hoped he might tell us something more encouraging than Dr. Alden's advice that I needed the dreaded "Whipple" surgery.

Things did not start out well. We had great difficulty finding Dr. Allendorf's office. This highlighted yet another frustrating experience we cancer patients are too often subjected to. The representative on the phone who made the appointment failed to tell us how difficult it was to find the doctor's office ... and nearby parking. It turned out to be so difficult, we had to call the doctor's office several times before finally locating the office and nearby parking.

When we did finally get to the doctor's office, I was tempted to complain but I resisted - especially since I felt irritable and cranky from hormones the NET tumors send out into the body. I

MY JOURNEY WITH NEUROENDOCRINE CANCER
What You Don't Know Can Kill You!

focused instead on a comforting thought - at least I was given the right appointment date and time! As other cancer patients can attest – this is not always how things work out.

I handed the receptionist my numerous lab reports and CDs, and in turn was given the usual mountain of papers and forms to complete and return. After filling them out ... we sat and waited ... and waited ... and waited. Long waits in doctors' waiting rooms is another frustrating quality-of-care routine that oncologists and staff put us cancer patients through.

It seems oncologists and their clerical staff are oblivious to the exceedingly difficult life we cancer patients live with. Quality-of-care issues that beg for improvement includes making sure appointments are made and communicated accurately, reducing excessive waiting times, improving the comfort of waiting areas, reducing the mountains of paperwork, improving the accuracy of billing statements, and more.

It is way past the time when oncologists should focus on such quality-of-care issues and make necessary improvements wherever possible. Oncologists may not always be able to cure the type of cancer we patients suffer with ... but they should be able to improve quality-of-care issues.

When Margie and I finally got to see Dr. Allendorf, it didn't take very long for us to realize he didn't hold neuroendocrine cancer in very high regard. Judging by his comments, I worried I might actually be one of the first neuroendocrine cancer patients he has treated. Since then, other NET cancer patients have shared how they had similar experiences with their doctors and oncologists. If the doctors and oncologists are not familiar with neuroendocrine cancer, they should tell us and perhaps refer us to other medical professionals. The knowledge and experience of the doctors and oncologists who treat us has a direct effect on our quality of life ... and can be the difference between life and death.

Dr. Allendorf began the consultation by reviewing his extraordinary experience in dealing with various cancers. It was very impressive to hear. Then he spoke about the neuroendocrine cancer.

"There are people who don't even know they have neuroendocrine cancer until after they have died from something else, and an autopsy discovers they had it. Since neuroendocrine cancer grows so slowly, Mr. Walsh, and the tumor you have is so small, you will likely die from something else. For that, you certainly do **NOT** need Whipple surgery!"

I then explained how another oncologist, Dr. Dmitri Alden, told us he had done over 2,500 Whipple surgeries, and that my case of neuroendocrine cancer was so serious, he strongly recommended I have the Whipple surgery as soon as possible.

Dr. Allendorf scoffed, "First of all, **I** have never heard of a Dr. Dmitri Alden ... and I seriously doubt he has ever done over 2,500 Whipple surgeries! If he did, I am sure I would have heard about it ... and I certainly have not!"

Looking past Margie and me, he called out to his two assistants sitting directly behind us.

"Have either of you ever heard of a Doctor Dmitri Alden?"

Both assistants replied, "No, they hadn't."

Turning back to me, Dr. Allendorf said, "Mr. Walsh, the small neuroendocrine tumor you have is very slow-growing, and is usually benign. It certainly is **NOT** something you should be worried about. You will likely outlive it and die from something else!"

I was surprised by Dr. Allendorf's cavalier attitude toward neuroendocrine cancer, and my condition in particular. I already knew - for all the reasons he stated - NET cancer is a very dangerous, sinister malignancy that cannot so easily be brushed off. Just ask families of NET cancer patients who died from it.

MY JOURNEY WITH NEUROENDOCRINE CANCER
What You Don't Know Can Kill You!

I told the doctor, "In spite of all that, doctor, the clinical fact remains that my NET tumor ... no matter how small it may be ... and no matter how slowly it may grow ... it can be ... as specifically happened in my case ... powerful enough to close my entire biliary system, and leave me in danger of dying!"

Judging by the expression on the doctor's face, the aggressive manner in which I said this was taken as confrontational. Dr. Allendorf appeared to take my remarks as a challenge to what he said. (It didn't help that this happened in the presence of his two assistants I heard giggling.)

Ignoring this, I persisted, "Dr. Allendorf ... **NOT EVERYONE** outlives neuroendocrine cancer? It is a sinister, incurable cancer that affects its victims in different ways ... and it DOES kill some of us!

"What's more ... it is not only the size of the tumor that matters ... and it is not only how slowly it grows that matters ... it is also about WHERE the tumor roots itself ... and how sick it makes the patient from the hormones the tumors give off!"

My words further annoyed Dr. Allendorf as he angrily rose up out of his chair, stomped over to the door of his office, and snapped, **"I have other patients in my waiting room who have real cancers! GOODBYE!"**

Margie and I were stunned by the doctor's sudden, unprofessional behavior.

We stopped at the door where I protested, "Doctor, I cannot believe you said that! That is so inappropriate!"

Dr. Allendorf simply stood there apparently trying to think of what to say in response. He apparently was not accustomed to being challenged by one of his patients ... especially in front of two staff members ... and a waiting room filled with "other patients who have real cancers."

As Margie and I walked past the people in the waiting room, I realized each one of them was suffering with some type of cancer. They, and the caregivers with them, looked so sad and troubled. I said a silent prayer for them.

On our drive home, Margie and I were discouraged - and offended - by Dr. Allendorf's words.

I wondered aloud, "How is it possible such a brilliant oncologist like Dr. Allendorf can be so poorly informed about neuroendocrine cancer ... and say something so insensitive? Rather than helping us, he wound up insulting us ... and wasted so much of our precious little time!"

It was beginning to sink in how many oncologists - even those with a good reputation - don't fully understand neuroendocrine cancer. In time, other NET cancer patients would share with us how they, too, suffered frustrating experiences at the hands of doctors and oncologists who had little understanding of NET cancer ... or how to treat it.

A NET cancer patient once told me, "Welcome to the club, Bob! Don't feel too badly, and try not to take the frustrations too personally. You are not alone, you know. Most people with NET cancer can tell you how they, too, suffer in similar ways."

The next stop on my journey with neuroendocrine cancer was an appointment on March 23, 2017 at Northwell Laboratories on East Main Street in Bay Shore, Long Island, New York. This is where I was able to use a prescription written by Dr. Dmitri Alden to have special blood and urine tests done to gauge what affect the neuroendocrine cancer was having in my body. I could not believe how many vials of blood they took.

Four days later, I was at Zwanger-Pesiri Radiology facility in Deer Park, Long Island where an ultrasound sonogram was done on my kidneys to determine what damage, if any, was being done

MY JOURNEY WITH NEUROENDOCRINE CANCER
What You Don't Know Can Kill You!

by the neuroendocrine cancer. Ultimately, this sonogram determined that my kidneys were okay.

Later that same day, I went to see Dr. Robert Turoff, a brilliant oncologist and general surgeon located in Bay Shore, New York. I wanted his advice on ways to treat neuroendocrine cancer. Dr. Turoff said the best advice he had was to seek oncologists with as much experience as possible dealing with neuroendocrine cancer.

"Do yourself a favor, Mr. Walsh. This cancer is soooo rare, you need to avoid oncologists who don't have specific knowledge and experience with it. If ultimately you find you do need Whipple surgery, I strongly recommend a colleague who is a surgeon at Mount Sinai Hospital in New York City. He is one of the top surgeons in the country when it comes to performing Whipple surgery."

I thanked Dr. Turoff for his advice and recommendations ... and prayed I would never have to use the surgeon he recommended to do the Whipple surgery.

The very next day, March 28, 2017, I went to the Northwell Imaging Laboratory in Bay Shore, New York where a DOTA-TATE[7] (Gallium 68) whole body CT/PET scan was conducted. The Gallium 68 is a unique contrast that can identify the presence of small NET tumors in the body.

Once again, a prescription by Dr. Dmitri Alden was used to have this unique CT/PET scan with Gallium 68 done. The goal was to gauge the physical extent of neuroendocrine cancer throughout my body. This procedure took several hours to complete.

My journey with neuroendocrine cancer those days was consumed with making one medical appointment after another ... attending one doctor's visit after another ... having one lab test

---

[7] **DOTA-TATE** (Gallium-68) is a contrast used to measure tumor density and whole body distribution via CT/PET imaging.

done after another … completing one pile of medical forms after another … keeping endless notes … trying to find more information about NET cancer … and explaining to family and friends what exactly was wrong with me. All aspects of my life had become consumed by my journey with neuroendocrine cancer.

Thank God I had my wife, Margie, family members and friends accompany me along my painful journey.

A later report produced by two Northwell pathologists independently confirmed the presence of a malignant neuroendocrine tumor on my ampulla of vater. The report stated, in part, "Somatostatin receptor bearing lesion in the ampulla, corresponding to biopsy-proven neuroendocrine tumor."

Although this summary was what I expected, it was still very depressing to read. The reality of having this unwanted, intrusive, deadly, incurable cancer sank in ever more deeply. What comforted me was the love and support of family and friends, and my faith in God. Every day, I prayed for fellow cancer patients, their loved ones, doctors and oncologists.

In particular, I prayed no other patient with an incurable cancer would ever hear a doctor say, "I have other patients with real cancers."

MY JOURNEY WITH NEUROENDOCRINE CANCER
What You Don't Know Can Kill You!

Chapter 9

DOCTOR EDWARD WOLIN

Shortly before I learned I had neuroendocrine cancer, the youngest of my seven sisters, Diana Walsh, was diagnosed with this same rare cancer.

Thank God, Diana is a strong, resilient individual. She is more like a daughter since my wife, Margie, and I, raised her along with my other four younger sisters when my parents died when the girls were very young. Mom died from breast cancer that had metastasized; Dad died from congenital heart disease. When my sisters were added to our own three children, we were like the "Waltons" in real life - one for every age problem!

Before the shock of having NET cancer wore off, Diana made an appointment in April 2017 for us to meet with the internationally renowned neuroendocrine cancer oncologist, Dr. Edward M. Wolin. Highly-esteemed by colleagues and patients alike, Dr. Wolin is one of the foremost leaders in the field.

Our first meeting took place in his office at the Montefiore Einstein Center for Cancer Care in the Bronx, New York. Within one year, however, Dr. Wolin was appointed director of Mount Sinai Hospital's group of medical scientists in New York City dedicated to the research and treatment of neuroendocrine cancer. Diana and I have since learned how this group of professionals are considered among the very best in the world.

When we read the formal announcement at the time of that appointment, Diana and I realized how incredibly fortunate we were to be among the first patients in Mount Sinai Hospital's program under Dr. Wolin's direction. Here is a copy of the announcement.

"**Edward M. Wolin, MD**, an internationally-renowned authority on neuroendocrine tumors, is Director of the Center for Carcinoid and

Neuroendocrine Tumors and Professor of Medicine, Hematology and Medical Oncology. He is the second director of the Center, which was founded by Richard P. Warner, MD, Professor of Medicine, Gastroenterology.

"The multi-disciplinary center features a robust research program with clinical trials aimed at finding the most effective treatments, including immunotherapy, biologic agents, targeted radiation therapy, and new approaches in molecular imaging for diagnosis. Dr. Wolin has pioneered innovative therapies with novel somatostatin analogs, mTOR[8] inhibitors, anti-angiogenic drugs, and peptide receptor radiotherapy.

"Prior to joining Mount Sinai, Dr. Wolin was Director of the Neuroendocrine Tumor Program at Montefiore Einstein Center for Cancer Care. Previously, he worked for more than two decades with Cedars-Sinai Medical Center in Los Angeles, where he founded and directed one of the largest carcinoid and neuroendocrine tumor programs in the country. Currently, Dr. Wolin serves as Co-Medical Director for the Carcinoid Cancer Foundation and is on the Carcinoid Cancer Research Grants Scientific Review Committee for the American Association for Cancer Research. He is a reviewer for numerous journals, including Journal of Clinical Oncology, Molecular Cancer Therapeutics, Clinical Cancer Research, and The Lancet Oncology.

"Certification: Medical Oncology, American Board of Internal Medicine.
Education: MD, Yale University School of Medicine.
Internship: Internal Medicine: Stanford University Hospital.
Residency: Internal Medicine, Stanford University Hospital.
Fellowship: Medical Oncology, Stanford University Hospital."

Prior to our first consultation with Dr. Wolin, he requested that we forward copies of all relevant health conditions and issues including and all lab reports. At our meeting, we were greatly

---

[8] **mTOR** - mTOR inhibitors are a class of drugs that regulate cellular metabolism, growth and proliferation by forming and signaling through two protein complexes, mTORC1 and mTORC2. The most established mTOR inhibitors are so-called rapalogs (rapamycin and its analogs) which have shown tumor responses in clinical trials against various tumor types. Studies suggest that mTOR inhibitors may have anticancer activity in many cancer types such as **neuroendocrine tumors**, breast cancer, hepatocellular carcinoma, renal cell carcinoma (RCC), sarcoma and large B-cell lymphoma.

MY JOURNEY WITH NEUROENDOCRINE CANCER
What You Don't Know Can Kill You!

impressed with Dr. Wolin's steady smile and easy, relaxed manner. To our great relief, he was also an excellent communicator who listened well and clearly answered our questions. When he reviewed our various health issues, he patiently listened to our many questions and concerns.

He then explained that Diana and I had what he called, "a rare familial form of neuroendocrine cancer."

"This type of cancer runs in your family," he stated. "All your siblings and children should be tested to see if any of them also have it. You two have quite a big job ahead of you but I assure you, I will do everything I can to assist you in communicating this to family members. It is very important that you do so."

True to his word over time, Dr. Wolin would be very helpful throughout our ongoing ordeal as we struggled to explain something as complex and mysterious as neuroendocrine cancer to family members. You imagine how difficult this was to achieve when even many doctors and oncologists do not fully understand it.

Doctor Wolin advised Diana, "You are going to require surgery to have the NET tumors removed. If I were you, Diana, I would not waste any time in getting this done. In fact, I wouldn't put off having surgery done longer than two, three months ... at the latest!"

Diana agreed, "Bob and I soon will be going to the National Institutes of Health (NIH) in Bethesda, Maryland. That's where I plan to have the surgery done."

Turning to me, Dr. Wolin said, "Yours is the rarest of rare forms of neuroendocrine cancer because of where the lesion is located. In particular, I recommend further tests be done before you decide whether or not to have the extensive 'Whipple' surgery to remove the tumor on your ampulla."

He stated how pleased he was that we were going to be part of Mount Sinai's program for neuroendocrine cancer, and NIH's program as well.

"NIH also has a dedicated team thoroughly familiar with neuroendocrine cancer … and they have the requisite equipment needed to run the special tests you both should have done."

Diana and I wasted no time in making an appointment to go to NIH in Bethesda, Maryland where intense testing would be done in late May 2017. Before this was to take place, however, my personal journey with neuroendocrine cancer was about to experience an unexpected encounter with the miraculous.

Chapter 10

"THE TUMOR IS GONE!"

These startling words were loudly exclaimed by my doctor setting the stage for one of the remarkable miracles I experienced on my extraordinary journey with neuroendocrine cancer. Allow me to share the details.

On April 17, 2017, I found myself lying on an operating table in a cold surgical room at St. Francis Hospital in Roslyn, Long Island, New York. Doctor Rajiv Bansal was about to conduct another endoscopy with EUS and ERCP. The goal this time was to determine how far the NET tumor located at the bottom of my common bile duct at the ampulla of vater had progressed since he first saw it there weeks before.

Prior to starting the procedure, Doctor Bansal explained once again, "Mr. Walsh, I am going to do my best to take out as much of the tumor as I can. This is very difficult and dangerous to do with a neuroendocrine tumor[9] because they root themselves down into the surrounding area … much like a tree roots itself into the ground. If I go too deep in trying to remove some of it, I might inadvertently puncture some of the highly-delicate surrounding tissue. This would create quite a serious emergency requiring far more extensive surgery.

"I promise you, I will do what I can to remove as much of the tumor as I can to give you more time. If this doesn't work … you might have to have the 'Whipple' surgery after all!"

While lying on the cold operating table, right after I finished praying, I looked up and saw a large clock hanging on the opposite

---

[9] **Neuroendocrine Tumor** - This tumor is one that forms from cells that release hormones into the blood in response to signals from the nervous system. Such a tumor is also called a NET, or "Carcinoid."

wall from where I was lying. I was quite amazed and thrilled to see the time was the same as the last procedure I had weeks earlier.

It was three o'clock ... the hour of Divine Mercy!

At that very moment, the whirling effects of the general anesthesia began to set in. As they did, I felt the benefit of many prayers and Masses said for me. They flowed down upon me ... and blanketed me like a huge, beautiful, spiritual comforter.

The last few seconds before I going completely out, I prayed, "Thank you, God ... and everyone who prayed for me."

The next thing I knew, I awoke in the recovery room with my wife, Margie, and my daughter, Peggie, standing on either side of my bed. Dr. Bansal soon appeared. Actually, he came rushing into the room and stood at the foot of my bed looking puzzled.

Catching his breath, he shouted, "The tumor is gone! There's nothing there now! Nothing! And all the damage I saw in your system weeks ago is also gone! Everything looks normal! I can't explain it."

Margie replied, "We can ... we prayed!"

The doctor smiled, "Just to be sure, I took many biopsies. I'll call you with the pathology report as soon as it comes in."

As quickly as he had rushed in, Dr. Bansal left. Margie, Peggie and I stared at each other ... thrilled by what we just heard. After a spontaneous giggle, we embraced, cried and heartily thanked God.

The doctor said the tumor was gone! The tumor was gone! As this good news spread among family and friends, I wondered if this meant the underlying cancer was also gone?

Days later, Dr. Bansal called with results of the biopsies he had taken. St. Francis Hospital pathologists confirmed the amazing news ... the cancerous neuroendocrine tumor on my ampulla of vater was gone. It literally vanished!

MY JOURNEY WITH NEUROENDOCRINE CANCER
What You Don't Know Can Kill You!

Doctors familiar with my condition could not explain how a tumor known to root itself downward like a tree, simply disappeared. Those familiar with what happened realized Doctor Bansal personally saw the cancerous tumor in my body only a few weeks earlier, and using special equipment, took color pictures of the lesion and took several biopsies which different pathologists later confirmed was, in fact, a malignant neuroendocrine tumor.

This time, Dr. Bansal stated in his surgical operating report there was no sign of significant pathology in the ampulla; no evidence of a remaining neuroendocrine tumor.

It was clear to me and everyone who prayed for me this was one of those miraculous times when God wanted to make sure everyone involved knew He had intervened. There was no mistake this time … God miraculously took take away the neuroendocrine tumor.

But to my dismay as I would later learn, God took away the tumor … but **NOT** the underlying cancer.

This particular endoscopy procedure unfortunately badly irritated the sensory nerves on the left side of my jaw. The pain I suffered was absolutely terrible. I offered up the pain for the holy souls in Purgatory as the extreme pain continued for a few weeks. Eventually, I had to go see an endodontist, Dr. Robert Shamul, Babylon, New York. He ran several tests which confirmed the pain was not coming from any of my teeth; they were fine. He surmised the pain was caused by the endoscopy I had on April 17th at St. Francis Hospital. He said it likely greatly irritated the highly sensitive nerves in my jaw.

"That is not uncommon. In time, the pain you are experiencing should subside; it's not permanent," he assured me.

A few days later, I received a call from Joanne Forbes, a Physician's Assistant at the National Institutes of Health (NIH) in Bethesda, Maryland. She informed me that my sister, Diana, and I had been accepted into NIH's research and treatment program as part of their familial study of neuroendocrine (NET) cancer. Their studies already indicated neuroendocrine cancer can run in families, and that my particular form of NET cancer is regarded is one of the rarest of the rare!

Before I could go to NIH, I first had to go in mid-May to see Dr. Strachovsky, Ophthalmologist. After running the usually extensive tests, he reported the wet macular degeneration in my right eye had become much worse. Accordingly, he anesthetized my right eye then administered the third injection of Avastin in the hope it might close up the bleeding capillaries in my right eye and thereby stop the bleeding.

MY JOURNEY WITH NEUROENDOCRINE CANCER
What You Don't Know Can Kill You!

Chapter 11

"WE MAY NOT BE ABLE TO SAVE YOUR SIGHT"

I had yet to wrap my mind around how to cope with the ravages of neuroendocrine cancer when I was hit with more disturbing news. On June 23, 2017, my ophthalmologist, Dr. Strachovsky, told me the special tests he ran showed the damage done to my right eye by wet macular degeneration had become much, much worse.

"I am sorry to tell you, Mr. Walsh, the Avastin medication we've been using is simply not working. I am afraid the damage done to your right eye is **NOT** reversible! If you want, we can try another, stronger medication called, 'Eylea,' at your next appointment."

I agreed but under the circumstances, I decided to get a second opinion so I went to see Dr. David Fastenberg, another highly regarded ophthalmologist and retina specialist at "LI Vitroretinal" in Hauppauge, New York.

After conducting a series of extensive tests, the doctor reported, "I fully agree with Dr. Strachovsky's diagnosis. Now you have to hope the sight in your left eye stays healthy and doesn't also develop wet macular degeneration. You realize, Mr. Walsh, if that happens ... you will be blind!"

Leaving this doctor's office, I felt overwhelmed by the weight of all that was happening to me. Before I allowed myself to go on a "pity party," however, I knew there were many other people in the world who were far worse off than I was so I resolved to continue offering all my sufferings and frustrations for the poor souls in Purgatory.

A few days later I went back to Dr. Strachovsky who ran the usual extensive tests on my right eye and said the macular degeneration had become even worse as he feared. He then injected my right eye for the first time with Eylea, the stronger medication. I hoped for the best but deep down inside, I sensed that - short of a miracle - I was eventually going to lose the sight in my right eye.

Besides praying God would spare me from the ravages of neuroendocrine cancer, I now also prayed He would spare me from complete blindness.

MY JOURNEY WITH NEUROENDOCRINE CANCER
What You Don't Know Can Kill You!

Chapter 12

NATIONAL INSTITUTES OF HEALTH (NIH)

On an early Sunday morning in June 2017, my sister, Diana, and I, two NET cancer patients, drove from Deer Park, Long Island to NIH's Clinical Center on Center Drive in Bethesda, Maryland. It took us more than seven grueling hours in surprisingly heavy traffic to make the trip. It should have taken us only five to six hours.

"We just can't catch a break, can we?" Diana and I both laughed at the same time.

When we finally arrived at NIH, we were greatly surprised

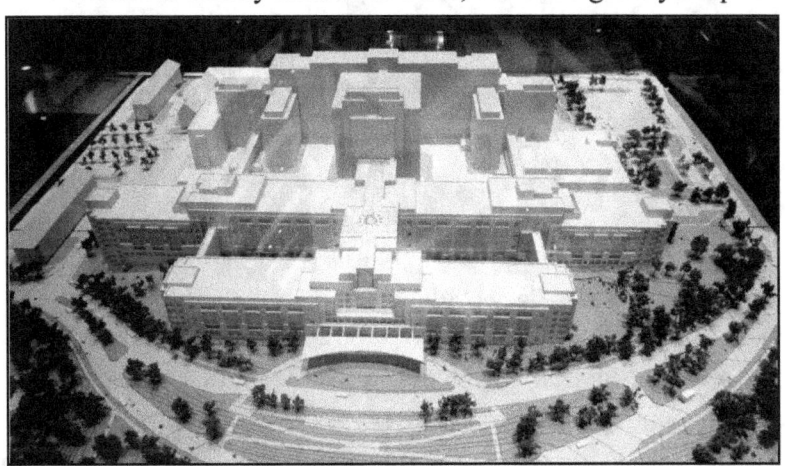

by the enormous size of NIH's hospital grounds as shown above. After going through NIH's impressive security checkpoint, we received patient passes and then proceeded directly to the Edmond J. Safra Family Lodge on the grounds. That is where we stayed until we were admitted to the NIH Hospital for comprehensive, weeklong medical testing and evaluations.

The Edmond J. Safra Family Lodge offers a picturesque, home-like place of respite for families whose loved ones receive care at NIH's Clinical Research Hospital. Patients from across

America and around the world visit NIH to participate as partners in medical discovery. God bless them all.

Built in the style of an early 1900 English arts and crafts manor, the Safra Lodge offers convenient, comfortable, complimentary accommodations for families and caregivers so they can be nearby when loved ones receive intensive medical research and treatment.

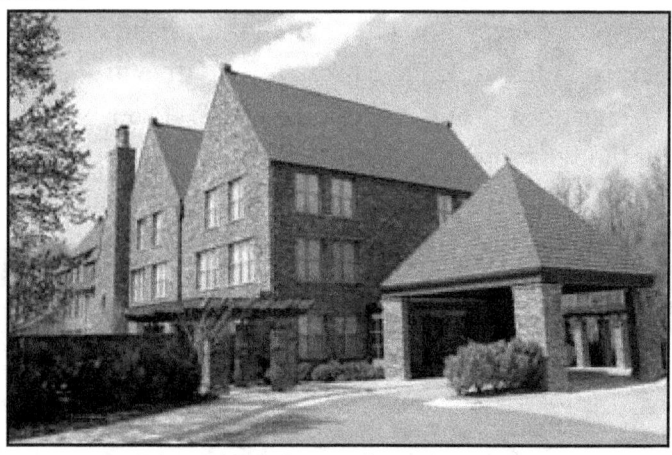

Edmond J. Safra Family Lodge at NIH

The following day, Diana and I were admitted to NIH's Clinical Center Hospital for the duration of our weeklong stay. Quite early that first day, we met the NIH team that would be studying us under the direction of Dr. Stephen A. Wank.

Dr. Wank began by warmly welcoming us and introducing himself and each member of his small team of special assistants. He clearly stated the goal of NIH's "protocol" (their reference to how the study is conducted) was to learn as much as they could about the very rare form of familial neuroendocrine cancer that Diana and I had. He explained that prior to our arrival at NIH, he and his team thoroughly reviewed all the records each of us had forwarded. This included all our medical records, CDs, lab reports, family medical history and much more.

MY JOURNEY WITH NEUROENDOCRINE CANCER
What You Don't Know Can Kill You!

Dr. Wank's assistant, Joanne Forbes, Physician's Assistant, explained how the protocol would be conducted including special blood, urine tests, X-rays, CT[10] scans, a MRI, F-Dopa CT/PET scan, Gallium 68 scan and more. She added how at the end of each day, the team would meet with us to review the results of each day's tests.

Throughout this initial presentation, Diana and I were given ample opportunity to ask questions. We were greatly impressed with how Dr. Wank and his team carefully listened and patiently provided clear, succinct information. Under the circumstances, this was quite comforting.

Precisely according to plan, over the course of the upcoming week, we were guided to the many test areas where each specific test was to be done within the vast NIH complex. As promised, Dr. Wank and his team came to our room each day and patiently, clearly explained the results of tests completed that day.

By the end of the week, Dr. Wank advised Diana that results of her tests clearly showed she had five (5) neuroendocrine tumors lined up right next to one another in the ileum of her small intestine!

It is important to note that all the blood and urine tests conducted by her doctors before Diana arrived at NIH, did not show any signs of neuroendocrine cancer! The only way she discovered she had NET tumors was through a routine colonoscopy that was conducted for other reasons!

Dr. Wank calmly stated, "Surgical removal of those tumors is strongly recommended ... and that it be done as soon as possible! The surgery can be done here at NIH by Dr. Jeremy Davis, a fine surgeon with a great deal of experience."

---

[10] **CT** - Also known as "computed tomography," uses computer-processed combinations of many Xray measurements taken at different angles to produce cross-sectional images (virtual "slices") of specific areas of a scanned object. This allows users to see inside the object without cutting. Other terms include computed axial tomography (CAT scan) and computer aided tomography.

After a short pause, he cautioned, "Wherever you choose to have the surgery done ... I don't think you should delay."

Diana assured him she would, in fact, proceed in having the needed surgery done at NIH as soon as arrangements could be made.

Turning to me, Dr. Wank informed me my test results showed the neuroendocrine tumor originally found on my ampulla of vater did, in fact, appear to be gone. He cautioned, however, there was some uncertainty involved.

"The F-Dopa CT/PET scan showed there is a pooling in the area of your ampulla of vater ... right where the tumor was originally located. The pathologist who analyzed your scan has many years of experience. His finding is that the pooling may, in fact, be caused by the physiological nature of your body in that area. However, he also clearly cautions that we cannot rule out the possibility that there may be a residual tumor located within that pooling! We just cannot be sure at this time ... so that area will require further ongoing monitoring.

"I also must tell you that the F-Dopa scan - and the MRI - both showed a neuroendocrine lesion is located in a lymph node on the left crus of your diaphragm close to your spine. It appears it metastasized there."

After a brief pause, he continued, "In fact, the CD you gave us of a CT/PET scan that was taken back in late 2009 showed that tumor was already there. Although this particular lesion was an active malignancy, it has not grown since 2009!"

After allowing me another moment to digest this disturbing news, Dr. Wank added, "You know, it is highly likely that you have many other - very small - neuroendocrine tumors located in other areas of your body. If there are, they are too small to be detected at this time."

MY JOURNEY WITH NEUROENDOCRINE CANCER
What You Don't Know Can Kill You!

I asked if it was possible these other "possible" NET tumors might be active despite being very small.

Dr. Wank said, "Well, yes; it is very possible."

Needless to say, I found this news surprising and devastating to hear. My sister, Diana, sitting next to me, actually appeared to be more upset than I was. For her benefit, I remained composed and tried not to show how alarmed I was to hear the disappointing news. The reality that this cancer might actually kill me sank in even deeper.

Searching for something, anything, to say to fill the uncomfortable silence hanging in the air, I blurted out, "Okay ... so what can I do about this, doctor? Why don't I just have the tumor in my diaphragm cut out?"

Wasting no time to respond, Dr. Wank bluntly snapped, "It's too late now! The cat is already out of the bag! The cancer has already spread! Besides ... it would be far too dangerous to try to remove it!"

I was taken aback by Dr. Wank's unexpectedly blunt, frank statement.

"Besides, it is so small," the doctor added, "a surgeon might not be able to find the lesion when he opens you up! It's so small; he might not be able to see it."

His straightforward blunt words, surprised everyone leading to yet another, terribly uncomfortable, awkward silence. Dr. Wank appeared to be waiting for me to say something ... or to ask another question.

Finally, I thought to ask, "Well, doctor, if surgery cannot be done ... what about chemo?"

Looking somewhat relieved, Dr. Wank nodded and said, "You could consider having synthetic Somatostatin analogue[11]

---

[11] **Analogue** – An analogue, also known as a chemical analogue, is something that is

treatments. Such analogue treatments are recommended by some oncologists in cases like yours where surgery is not an option to remove neuroendocrine tumors. They are administered by injection on a monthly or other periodic basis."

After a pause, he added, "Some oncologists believe synthetic analogue treatments have the effect of slowing down the growth and spread of neuroendocrine cancer in the body. At the same time, they are believed to lessen the side effects of carcinoid syndrome. However, I should tell you, there is no clear clinical evidence as yet to support such beliefs.

"A decision to use a somatostatin analogue to deal with neuroendocrine cancer comes with a number of significant risks. These include the possibility that analogue treatments might cause formation of gallstones, cause changes to your blood sugar possibly resulting in diabetes, slow down your heart rate, and possibly cause hypertension. These are all serious issues for you to consider when thinking of having synthetic somatostatin analogue treatments. The decision is yours, Mr. Walsh."

I asked, "Given my specific condition with neuroendocrine cancer, do you think I should try synthetic somatostatin injections?"

Dr. Wank shrugged his shoulders and carefully replied, "I just don't know if a somatostatin analogue would be helpful for you, Mr. Walsh. Everyone's body is an entirely different environment. What works for one person, may not work for another. It's entirely up to you, Mr. Walsh. You must decide."

I thanked the doctor for his candor, and said, "I obviously have a lot of research to do to learn as much as I can about this cancer ... and the synthetic Somatostatin analogue treatments."

---

similar or comparable to something else either in general or some specific detail.

MY JOURNEY WITH NEUROENDOCRINE CANCER
What You Don't Know Can Kill You!

"In conclusion," Dr. Wank said, "we think it would be a good idea for you to have another endoscopy performed in a few months to see what ... if any ... changes there might be. Also, we'd like you to return to NIH every six months for us to conduct our full series of tests to monitor your neuroendocrine cancer ... and hopefully ... learn more about the rare form you have."

I asked who he thought should do the endoscopy.

Dr. Wank confidently replied, "It makes a lot of sense for you to have the same gastroenterologist, Doctor Bansal, who did the recent endoscopies on you, do the next one. After all, he was the one who was in there already and saw everything. He, logically, would be the one most familiar with your condition."

With that, Dr. Wank and his team wished us well and departed. Diana and I sat there in silence for a few moments allowing all the disturbing news each of us received to sink in. Amusingly, both of us shrugged our shoulders at the same time and chuckled.

Diana then said what was going through both our minds, "Oh, well, all that really, really stinks."

In reply, I said something our father, Patrick Victor Walsh, must have said a thousand times over the years, "You know, when the going gets tough ... the tough get going!"

After a quick laugh, we hugged.

Just then, a priest in full clerical garb entered the room and gleefully introduced himself, "Hi, folks, I am Monsignor Dominic Ashkar. I am the Catholic Chaplain here at NIH. I understand the two of you are Catholic. Is this a good time to visit?"

Diana and I giggled as I answered, "Wow ... does a rabbit have ears? Talk about perfect timing, Father ...this is a **VERY GOOD TIME** to visit! Diana and I just received some pretty disturbing news."

God obviously knew just the right time to send a Catholic priest into our midst to reassure us. What a tremendous comfort it was to have this warm, gentle man of God standing right there in our midst.

After polite introductions, Father Dominic listened to our plight with neuroendocrine cancer and then offered soothing words of understanding and encouragement. To our delight, Father told us he had Holy Communion with him!

"Would you like to receive?" he asked.

Diana and I were so overjoyed, we could only nod yes. Father Dominick reached into his jacket pocket and reverently retrieved a blessed pyx[12] containing the Eucharist. After saying a few prayers, Father gave Diana and me the sacred Host. The three of us then stood there in silence as warm, gentle rays of the sun streamed in upon us through the large windows. What a holy, special moment. For the moment, all was well.

---

[12] A **pyx** or **pix** (Latin) is a small round container used in Roman Catholic, Old Catholic and **Anglican** Churches to carry the consecrated host (**Eucharist**) to those who are sick or otherwise unable to come to church to receive **Holy Communion**.

Chapter 13

"A DEFINITE MAYBE"

Armed with a greater understanding of neuroendocrine cancer from the week I spent at NIH's Clinical Center (and the independent online research I was able to conduct), I went to see Dr. Rajiv Bansal, gastroenterologist, in his Lake Success, Long Island office.

Dr. Bansal began by telling my wife, Margie, and me that he had thoroughly reviewed all of NIH's report of findings, "I fully agree with NIH that the NET tumor I personally saw on your ampulla of vater weeks ago appears to be gone."

"I don't understand," Margie complained, "What do you mean, 'it **APPEARS** to be gone? Either the tumor is gone … or it isn't. Which is it? Is it gone or not?"

To our utter amazement, Dr. Bansal replied, "In terms of whether or not the lesion is gone, all I can tell you at this time is that it is … *A DEFINITE MAYBE!*"

Margie and I were more confused than ever.

Seeing our frustration, Dr. Bansal clarified, "Try to understand … the 'F-Dopa' test NIH ran did NOT show the presence of a residual tumor. However, it **DID SHOW** there was some 'pooling' in the area where I originally saw the tumor located."

"So what does that mean?" I demanded to know.

"What it means is this … there is no certainty at this time as to whether or not **SOME** of the NET tumor may still be there on your ampulla of vater! That's why I said, 'It is a definite maybe!' That is perhaps the reason you should consider beginning Sandostatin or Lanreotide somatostatin analogue treatments as a precaution."

Then, in keeping with what Dr. Wank said, Dr. Bansal added, "There's no clear evidence that synthetic somatostatin analogue treatments, in fact, slow down the growth and or the spread of neuroendocrine cancer. Moreover, such treatments do come with serious side-effects including damage to the gallbladder from formation of gallstones, changes to your blood sugar possibly leading to diabetes, damage to heart valves, and possibly leading to hypertension."

In terms of the next step, Dr. Bansal reiterated the last recommendation made by Dr. Wank at NIH, "I agree with Dr. Wank that you should consider having a follow-up endoscopy in a few months to gauge the progress of the neuroendocrine cancer. Would you like me to schedule you for another endoscopy?"

"I can tell you, there is no **'definite maybe'** about that," I joked. "Yes, please go ahead and make the necessary arrangements for you to do a follow-up endoscopy on me in a few months."

Chapter 14

DOCTOR GROSSLY INEPT

In late June 2017, I began monthly treatments by an oncologist on Long Island, New York. This doctor had been recommended to me by a fellow NET cancer patient who said the doctor was quite knowledgeable in treating patients with neuroendocrine cancer. After eight months of treatment, misinformation and injury at this doctor's hands, it was apparent he wasn't as qualified as he thought … and as I had hoped.

I have to assume this doctor meant well but considering the terrible experiences I suffered at his hands, I will not use his real name. Instead, I will refer to him as "Dr. Grossly Inept" because that is the name that best describes his medical capabilities in terms of neuroendocrine cancer.

With offices on Long Island, Dr. Grossly Inept presents himself as an oncologist with an expertise including diagnosis and treatment of neuroendocrine cancer. Unfortunately, this doctor turned out to be living proof of the saying, "a little knowledge can be a very dangerous thing!"

Other NET cancer patients later told me that my painful, frustrating experiences with this doctor were not really all that unusual for NET cancer patients. Many had suffered in similar ways with their doctors and oncologists. In fact, some shared how they suffered in far worse ways. Clearly, this should serve as a warning to other patients with neuroendocrine cancer to be sure the doctors and oncologists treating them have actual experience treating our rare cancer.

My experiences with Dr. Grossly Inept are a good, sad example. Although he was highly recommended to me, what follows are some of the more painful events I suffered.

A good place to begin is at my very first visit, I filled out the usual countless forms and handed them back to the receptionist along with my Medicare and AARP Plan K supplemental health insurance coverage cards. With my wife, Margie, at my side, I asked the receptionist to please confirm whether or not my health insurance coverage was acceptable as "in network" and that it was sufficient to cover the doctor's various fees.

Like most cancer patients, I was worried that the related medical costs might exceed my insurance coverage and ability to pay. I was especially concerned because Margie and I heard that treatments for NET cancer were very, very expensive - in fact, running in the many thousands of dollars in uncovered fees.

I told the receptionist, "I have heard treatment costs for my type of cancer can be very, very high. If my health insurance coverage is not sufficient to fully cover the costs, I can upgrade my AARP supplemental insurance coverage from Plan K to another plan that will more fully cover related costs."

I added, "In fact, depending on how high the uncovered costs are, I may decide NOT to have any treatments at all by Dr. Grossly Inept."

The receptionist said she understood then carefully reviewed each of my health insurance cards. She said she was familiar with the type of health insurance I had and could assure me my health insurance was in-network and was sufficient to cover Dr. Grossly Inept's various costs.

Over the following eight months, the doctor assured Margie and me a number of times that all the related costs were covered by my Medicare and AARP Plan K supplemental health insurance coverage.

We distinctly recall him saying, "Many of my other patients have the same insurance so I know everything will be covered. You won't owe a cent!"

MY JOURNEY WITH NEUROENDOCRINE CANCER
What You Don't Know Can Kill You!

Unfortunately for me, I didn't get such assurances in writing. Eight months later, I would find out Dr. Inept was not correct. It was at that time that he actually admitted during a recorded telephone call to my home that neither he nor his staff ever bothered to actually confirm whether or not my health insurance was sufficient to fully cover his treatment costs! He said they just assumed it was! They just assumed it was.

This, by the way, included the very expensive Sandostatin analogue treatments he administered to me over the eight months!

By the time finally he did check the sufficiency of my applicable health insurance, he discovered there was more than $3,200 in costs not fully covered by my Medicare and AARP Plan K supplemental coverage! In this recorded message, Dr. Inept outrageously said that he would **NOT** continue treating me until I paid him all of the money owed!

Allow me to say that again. Dr. Inept would **NOT** continue treating me, **a patient with an incurable cancer,** until I paid him all of the $3,200 owed! Mind you, my insurance coverage had already, in fact, paid him many thousands of dollars in his fees!

I, family members and other NET cancer patients were absolutely stunned that Dr. Inept, an oncologist treating me - a patient sick with incurable neuroendocrine cancer - stopped all further treatments of me because some of his fees were not covered due to his misjudgment of my insurance coverage!

This was especially disturbing given the fact that the doctor admitted on the same recorded telephone call that his fees were not fully covered because he and his staff never checked to see if my applicable insurance was sufficient. They just **assumed** it was!

To this day, I still find it so difficult to understand how an oncologist, any medical professional, can so cold-heartedly, immediately stop treating me, a patient sick with an incurable cancer, simply because of a little money owed! How terribly sad.

In addition, by misinforming me regarding his fees and the lack of sufficient insurance coverage, Dr. Inept denied me the ability to choose whether or not I, in fact, wished to incur such expensive treatments. In addition, I could also have chosen to add additional health insurance coverage if I only knew what I had was not fully sufficient to cover all cancer treatment fees.

Moreover, I later learned applicable laws do not permit a doctor to discontinue treating a patient because of non-payment of fees <u>unless the doctor does the following</u>:

- The doctor must continue treating the patient for thirty (30) days after proper notice; and,
- The doctor must assist the patient in finding another physician.

Dr. Grossly Inept certainly did not do any of the above. What he did do was to inhumanely cut me off from all further treatments. Other NET cancer patients later told me that the manufacturer of Sandostatin, Novartis Pharmaceutical, one of the medicines used to treat neuroendocrine cancer, has a charitable program to cover costs not covered by a patient's insurance! All that Novartis requires is for the oncologist to submit a simple form to Novartis. Neither Dr. Inept nor his staff ever did so.

To make matters even more painful. I later discovered that Dr. Inept and his staff were actually well-known to Novartis Pharmaceutical and were well aware of the Novartis charitable program. It turns out the doctor and his staff did not submit the necessary form to Novartis on my behalf because they didn't think it was needed!

Despite even this, the doctor's stated in his telephone message, "It is your responsibility, not mine, to make sure your insurance is sufficient to cover all costs. You must pay the uncovered fees and until you do, I am cannot treat you any further!"

MY JOURNEY WITH NEUROENDOCRINE CANCER
What You Don't Know Can Kill You!

Afterward, I appealed to Novartis Pharmaceutical and asked the company under the circumstances to cover the uncovered fees under its charitable program. Their response stunned me.

Novartis representatives cold-heartedly told me, "There is nothing we can do, Mr. Walsh, since the doctor did not submit the necessary form during your eight months of treatment with Sandostatin in 2017!"

I appealed to their sense of "understanding, compassion and consideration" given the fact that Dr. Inept readily admitted that he and his staff knew about the program but did not submit the forms.

I pleaded, "Given the spirit of Novartis' charitable program - and under the extenuating circumstances involved, can't Novartis reconsider and cover the uncovered costs."

I received the same dispassionate reply, "I am sorry, there is nothing Novartis can do when our form is not properly completed or submitted during the same year as treatments with Sandostatin!"

How sad. Had I known this is how Novartis treats patients with neuroendocrine cancer who use their Sandostatin medicine, I would have chosen the alternative medicine called Lanreotide which is manufactured by a different pharmaceutical company.

When my wife, Margie, and I first met the doctor, we could never have imagined him capable of such uncaring, unprofessional behavior. Allow me to take you back to our very first meeting with Dr. Grossly Inept.

At first, Dr. Inept appeared rather pleasant and friendly. He spent a great deal of time thoroughly reviewing his experience in diagnosing and treating neuroendocrine cancer. We were impressed at first but after a while, it seemed a little too much like he was bragging. But I gave him the benefit of the doubt until he actually complained about how he had to review "the many medical records, scans and lab reports you sent to me prior to this first consult!"

Wow! In retrospect, that perhaps should have put me on alert but I was desperate to find a qualified oncologist who was familiar with neuroendocrine cancer.

Following this inappropriate comment about the volume of my related medical information, the doctor asked for a verbal summary of my experience with neuroendocrine cancer - including current symptoms. I provided the following information as best I could recall:

- What happened when a neuroendocrine tumor in the bottom of my common bile duct at the ampulla closed my digestive system four months earlier;
- How I unintentionally lost more than 15 pounds during the prior several weeks; and,
- How I had been experiencing ongoing, intermittent deep red flushing on my face.

Oddly, before commenting on my review, the doctor asked what I did for a living before I retired. I told him I worked as an international banking executive for many years on Wall Street. Having asked me about my career, I fully expected he might ask some questions but he didn't say a word.

Instead, he said, "All your records, scans and lab reports clearly indicate you have neuroendocrine cancer."

I thought to myself, "Okay, thank you, doctor. But I already know that. Why don't you tell me something I don't know about neuroendocrine cancer ... and what I can do about it?!"

The doctor oddly silently sat there, staring blankly at us. This made me feel so uncomfortable I tried to encourage some helpful comments from him.

I said, "Dr. Stephen Wank, Director of research for neuroendocrine cancer at NIH stated there is clinical evidence now to show this cancer can run in families! In fact, Dr. Wank strongly

MY JOURNEY WITH NEUROENDOCRINE CANCER
What You Don't Know Can Kill You!

recommended that each of my five sisters, one brother and three children all be tested to see if any of them also have neuroendocrine cancer."

These words clearly perked up Dr. Inept as he eagerly volunteered, "I can run blood and urine tests for everyone in your family, Mr. Walsh. If these tests come back negative, that is sufficient to indicate they do NOT have neuroendocrine cancer."

I did not know at the time but Dr. Inept's words about the sufficiency of blood and urine tests **were absolutely not correct** to rule out the presence of neuroendocrine cancer! In fact, my younger sister, Diana Walsh, recently had perfectly normal blood and urine tests when at the same time a colonoscopy identified five (5) malignant neuroendocrine lesions in her ileum!

Dr. Grossly Inept went on to explain that I should consider receiving monthly injections of a synthetic somatostatin analog as NIH had recommended. He said there was a choice of Sandostatin or Lanreotide.

He added, "The jury is out on just how effective either of these are in terms of slowing down the cancer. To date, there is no clear clinical evidence to support this. What's more, both can have adverse effects on the gallbladder and other areas so we run tests every month to watch for detrimental. Each analogue appears to be equally effective ... but I find many patients tolerate Sandostatin better. The choice is yours, Mr. Walsh. I can administer either one."

I replied, "That's helpful to know, doctor but I am concerned about the related costs. Dr. Wank told me the injections can be very, very expensive, in fact, running in the thousands of dollars per injection. Accordingly, I don't want to get these injections unless I know they are covered by my health insurance. If my health insurance coverage isn't sufficient to cover the costs, I do not want to have any."

Dr. Grossly Inept asked what insurance I had. When I told him I had Medicare and AARP Plan K supplemental insurance, he smiled and assured me, "you have nothing to worry about; everything is covered. You won't owe anything."

With that assurance - and in light of the fact that I had an incurable malignant cancer - I decided to proceed with the Sandostatin treatments.

Dr. Grossly Inept explained that Sandostatin must be injected into a muscle; it cannot be administered via IV. Accordingly, he proceeded to inject me with a three-inch needle filled with Sandostatin 30 mg. He plunged the needle straight into the muscle! The buttock's cheek with a large muscle is the safest place to inject the three-inch needle. NET cancer patients refer to this Sandostatin injection as the "**Butt Dart**.")

The pain of the injection was nasty followed by a long-lasting, deep ache in my right buttock muscle. The pain extended all the way down my right leg. For the following seven to ten days, I felt like I had a case of the flu including nausea, extreme fatigue, chills, headache, and stool that consistently floated high in the water, and was light tan in color.

The "Butt Dart" and its resultant side effects were terrible but like other patients with an incurable cancer, I realized I didn't have much choice if I wanted to survive the NET cancer monster growing inside me.

Chapter 15

NIH's SURGICAL KNIGHT IN ARMOR DOCTOR JEREMY DAVIS

During the first week in August 2017, my wife, Margie, and I drove with my sister, Diana Walsh, to the National Institutes of Health (NIH), in Bethesda, Maryland where she was scheduled for laparoscopic surgery remove five (5) neuroendocrine tumors from her ileum.

We prayed the rosary asking God to bless the efforts of the surgeon, Dr. Jeremy L. Davis, and his assistants. Dr. Davis is a brilliant surgeon at NIH who was working in concert with NIH's clinical research and treatment program for neuroendocrine cancer.

The morning of the surgery, I accompanied Diana into the pre-surgical area, and encouraged her that this was finally a time for healing. Although understandably nervous, we were impressed with how well organized the many doctors and nurses were who were part of Diana's NIH surgical team.

Just before Diana was to be taken directly to the operating room, a surgeon marched into the area and barked out several orders - the last of which was quite aggressive as she addressed the entire surgical team.

She snapped, "I want to know which one of you has the Octreotide ready in case it is needed."

When no one immediately answered, she said combatively, "Well ... unless someone shows me the Octreotide right now ... this surgery is NOT going to take place!"

With that, there was a scramble of doctors and nurses running off to apparently to find the Octreotide! Within only a few minutes, an operating room nurse rushed into our area holding a bag of Octreotide for the surgeon to see.

"All right," she snapped, "That's what I needed to see! Listen up, guys, whenever we conduct surgery on a neuroendocrine patient, we must have Octreotide in the operating room with us in case it is needed!

"What do you say we get this pretty lady into the operating room before the day ends!"

Diana and I were amused - and greatly encouraged - by this unrehearsed last minute episode. We had only recently learned that the impact of surgery on a NET cancer patient under general anesthesia can sometimes have a dangerous - even fatal - effect on the patient's heart. If this happens during surgery, the doctors must have Octreotide immediately available - ready to administer to the patient right away. Having it there - if needed - is critical to the well-being, and, in some cases, survival of the patient.

After the surgery, Dr. Davis came out smiling and looking quite pleased as he told Margie and me that the surgery went well as expected. He confirmed that Diana did have five NET tumors virtually side-by-side in her ileum.

He reassured us, "I was able to remove the tumors without complications; I fully expect she will recover nicely."

After thanking him, Margie and I held hands and said a prayer of thanksgiving.

During the first day following surgery, Diana did so well, she was able to get up and walk around the hospital floor several times. The second day, however, was a different story. She was deathly ill and vomited several times. One of the doctors on her surgical team came to administer medications but nothing seemed to work! It took two full days before she was able to get past the tremendous pain and nausea but thank God, she eventually began to feel a little better.

Before we left NIH, we were so pleased that Monsignor Dominic Ashkar came to Diana's room to visit her. He brought

Holy Communion for us and prayed along with us. His mere presence was so comforting and reassuring. What a blessing he is for all the patients there at NIH.

After that long, tough week at NIH recovering from the surgery, Diana stayed with Margie and me in Deer Park, Long Island before returning to her home in upstate New York.

BOB WALSH

Chapter 16

TRYING TO SAVE MY SIGHT

At the next check-up on my eyesight on August 7, 2017, Dr. Strachovsky ran his usual tests to determine if the use of Eylea medication was able to slow down the gradual loss of sight in my right eye.

It didn't. In fact, the doctor said things had become even worse. The wet macular degeneration was relentlessly advancing … and destroying the sight in my right eye. Despite this discouraging news, I decided to have at least one more injection of Eylea. Thanks to Dr. Strachovsky's expertise, I barely felt any discomfort in once again having a needle stuck into my right eye.

Before I left, I asked if the doctor was aware of any connection between wet macular degeneration and neuroendocrine cancer. His said no, he wasn't aware of any. Given the sinister nature of neuroendocrine cancer, perhaps that is good news.

BOB WALSH

MY JOURNEY WITH NEUROENDOCRINE CANCER
What You Don't Know Can Kill You!

Chapter 17

"YOU LOOK SO GOOD!"

At my next monthly appointment with Dr. Grossly Inept, I told him how the first two months of Sandostatin (30 mg.) injections left me feeling as if I had a bad case of the flu - for up to two weeks after the injection. The misery included non-stop headache, nausea, lethargy, facial flushing and stool that was light tan in color and floated on the water surface.

Dr. Inept ignored what I said ... except for facial flushing. "You don't have facial flushing," he said gruffly.

Puzzled, I said, "Doctor, you don't know what my facial complexion normally looks like so how can you say I don't have facial flushing? My complexion is usually white as a ghost! The reddish coloring you see on my face is **NOT** the way I have looked most of my life!"

Margie confirmed my comments, "Doctor, don't you see all the reddish coloring on Bob's face? I can tell you that is **NOT** normal for him."

In a moment of breath-taking stupidity, Dr. Inept pompously blurted out, "Well, you may think so, but I don't see it. Given my experience with neuroendocrine cancer, I have to say your coloring looks perfectly normal to me! In fact, **you look so good!**"

As he sat there smiling smugly nodding his head up and down, I thought, "I cannot believe the doctor just said that! How can he possibly disagree with us about something so obvious as the deep red facial flushing I have?"

I don't think I will ever forget his words ... and the silly expression on his face. I worried then that I was dealing with an oncologist who doesn't listen to his patients, and doesn't accept what patients tell him about important issues such as symptoms.

This was followed by a disturbing thought - perhaps he is really not all that not familiar with neuroendocrine cancer and its symptoms. Or maybe he's just not very smart.

I began to worry about continuing treatments with Dr. Grossly Inept but I realized I needed a doctor who could administer the Sandostatin injections. So why not stay with him ... regardless of how grossly inept he appeared to be?

Margie closed this exchange by reminding Dr. Grossly Inept that facial flushing is why some people call neuroendocrine cancer the "good-looking cancer!" Dr. Grossly Inept ignored her comment as he simply rose up from his chair and left the room. When he returned, he held a three-inch needle to administer the Sandostatin injection. He promptly jammed the needle straight into my buttock. That was my third injection up to that time in 2017.

As usual, over the following two weeks, I felt as if I had a bad case of the flu with wicked, unrelenting painful symptoms including headache, nausea, chills and stool that floated on the water's surface and was consistently light tan in color.

And yes ... I did continue to experience **facial flushing.**

Chapter 18

THE "WAIT AND SEE" TREATMENT PLAN

On September 11, 2017, Dr. Rajiv Bansal, conducted another endoscopy on me - the third one in 2017. This time, the procedure was done without the necessity of EUS or ERCP at North Shore Hospital in Manhasset, Long Island, New York.

In the recovery room afterward, Dr. Bansal told my wife, Margie, my daughter, Peggie, and me that everything looked perfectly okay.

"I did not see anything that looked suspicious but I took pictures and thoroughly biopsied the entire area. As soon as I get the pathology report on the biopsies in a few days, I will call you with the results. If the biopsies come back negative - as I expect they will - then your treatment plan is going to be a **'wait and see'** strategy. That is what is usually done in cases like yours."

It was such a relief to hear the doctor say he didn't find anything new, but I wondered how could recommend I take a "wait and see" approach with a deadly cancer?

In time, I would learn from other NET cancer patients that this is the same advice their doctors and oncologists gave them as well. Wait and see ... wait and see ... wait and see.

When some NET cancer patients did wait and see ... the neuroendocrine cancer they had certainly did **NOT** follow the same advice. For several unfortunate NET cancer patients, the neuroendocrine cancer they had spread unchallenged resulting in terrible pain and suffering ... and for some, death.

BOB WALSH

Chapter 19

THE SIGHT IN MY RIGHT EYE IS GONE!

On September 18, 2017 and October 5, 2017, I saw Dr. Strachovsky, Ophthalmologist, at his office. After running extensive diagnostic tests, the doctor said the wet macular degeneration condition in my right eye had become much worse despite the three Eylea injections. The bleeding had formed scar tissue on the retina causing blindness.

"At this point," Dr. Strachovsky said dramatically, "I don't think further injections will do any good. There is nothing more we can do to save the sight in your right eye. The ongoing plan for you must be to monitor your good eye, the left one, to see if it develops wet macular degeneration.

"Let's hope it stays healthy," he said optimistically.

All I could think at the time was, "Wow ... the sight in my right eye is gone! Is this onslaught of bad news ever going to end?"

After I finished feeling sorry for myself, I renewed my ongoing resolution to offer all my sufferings up for the holy souls in Purgatory. At least that way, my sufferings would not go to waste.

"Thank God," I thought, "I still have sight in my left eye ... at least for now."

BOB WALSH

Chapter 20

DOCTOR GROSSLY INEPT STRIKES AGAIN!

On September 20, 2017, at the monthly scheduled appointment with Dr. Grossly Inept, I explained how the Sandostatin still made me sick for over a week following the injection. As with prior appointments, Dr. Grossly Inept ignored what I said and focused instead on my comment about having facial flushing.

"You don't have any sign of facial flushing," he argued as he had in the past. "If you had facial flushing from the neuroendocrine cancer, you would have a much brighter color than what you have!"

I didn't see the point in debating this with him so, instead, I asked, "Doctor, what about the other symptoms I have?"

"You obviously think the unpleasant things you are experiencing are from the injections. If they are ... and I am NOT saying they are ... some patients report the symptoms become more tolerable over time."

Dr. Inept then quickly changed the subject and had the audacity to complain that I had been saying since my first visit that I and other members of my family had the condition called hemochromatosis.

"What makes you think you and other family members have hemochromatosis? I haven't seen any clinical evidence of it."

Here he goes again, I lamented to myself.

"Doctor, on the very first day I saw you, I personally handed you a copy of a lab report that clinically confirmed I have both gene mutations of Hereditary Hemochromatosis, H63D and C262Y. That report and other lab statements are already in your files!"

"Oh, well, I'll have to check it," was his awkward reply.

Prior to giving me this month's Sandostatin 30 mg injection, I received an injection of vitamin B12 in my right shoulder. He then quickly went about getting the three-inch needle with Sandostatin, and wickedly stabbed it directly into my left buttock muscle. This was the fourth such injection in 2017. Once again, over the following 10 to 14 days, I felt like I had symptoms of the flu including headache, nausea, chills and stool that floated on the water's surface and was consistently light tan in color.

And yes … I still had occasional facial flushing.

Chapter 21

ST. ELIZABETH'S PARISH

On the night of October 16, 2017, I went to St. Elizabeth's Parish in Huntington, Long Island, New York where I was asked to give a talk on one of the very popular books I had written and published, "My Life of Miracles."

The evening began with recitation of the rosary in church. Afterward, everyone went to the large adjoining meeting room to hear my comments. During my talk, I spoke about how God had miraculously intervened many times over the course of my 72 years of life. Clearly, one of the highlights of my presentation was when I shared how I had recently learned I had an incurable, malignant cancer called neuroendocrine cancer.

"Earlier that momentous year, I had been diagnosed with this rare, incurable malignancy. During an endoscopic procedure, Dr. Bansal at North Shore University Hospital saw a deadly tumor located in the bottom of my common bile duct right at my ampulla of vater. The tumor was small but it was powerful enough to block and close off my digestive system. The doctor took color pictures of the tumor and did several biopsies. Later, pathologists at North Shore Hospital confirmed the tumor was a malignant NET lesion.

"Several weeks later, Doctor Bansal went back in to remove as much of the tumor as he could in an effort as he said, "to give you a little more time to live."

What happened utterly astonished him. The deadly tumor had literally disappeared! God took away the life-threatening tumor that had been blocking my digestive system ... but God did NOT take away the underlying cancer!"

After I completed this talk, a tearful woman accompanied by a few family members and friends came up to me and emotionally said, "My prayers were answered tonight in hearing you openly talk about having neuroendocrine cancer! I have been praying that God would send someone my way who also has neuroendocrine cancer.

"This was not so much for my benefit as it was for my family and friends. You see, it has been very difficult for them to believe I had some mysterious, unheard of rare cancer."

Stepping forward, she gave me a big hug and added, "My feelings of frustration and depression were lifted tonight with every word you said about 'NET' cancer!"

A family member standing nearby stepped up and whispered, "Me, too!"

MY JOURNEY WITH NEUROENDOCRINE CANCER
What You Don't Know Can Kill You!

Chapter 22

MISHAPS AT NIH

My sister, Diana, and I drove seven hours from Long Island, New York, to the National Institutes of Health (NIH) in Bethesda, Maryland for our next round of research and treatment for the neuroendocrine cancer each of us had. The schedule was to run from November 13, 2017 to November 17, 2017.

This was my second visit to NIH in 2017 where multiple tests were to be done as part of their ongoing study of the rare neuroendocrine cancer that runs in our family (familial cancer.) Under the direction of Dr. Stephen A. Wank, NIH's "protocol" included special blood and urine tests, various scans (an MRI, two PET/CT scans - one with Gallium-68 contrast, the other with F-DOPA contrast), and a CT scan with iodine contrast.

On Tuesday, November 14, 2017, I went by myself from my room located on the fifth floor in NIH's hospital to a special department located on another floor where a phlebotomist inserted a catheter IV into the top of my right hand. This was done so that contrast could later be injected through the catheter for several planned scans. I later learned this catheter was NOT supposed to be placed in my hand for the CT imaging. For the CT scan, it was only supposed to be placed in my forearm. I would later find out why.

When I returned to my hospital room, a nurse handed me two large bottles of Lumen to drink before going down to the CT imaging area on the first floor. Lumen is barium liquid that helps clear the abdomen for the type of scans to be done. Later at the appointed time, I went down to the CT imagining department on the first floor. There I joined other patients waiting to have a scan done. Like the others, I changed my clothes and put on a hospital gown. It was so incredibly cold in this area that I and other patients there were given warm blankets while we sat and waited for a scan to be done.

When it was my turn, I was led into a large room where a CT machine was located. As instructed, I laid down on a narrow table that was then moved inside the CT device. At some point, the CT technician told me he was injecting an iodine contrast into the catheter IV located on the top of my right hand. After he injected the iodine contrast, he quickly rushed away so he could then operate the CT machine from an area about ten feet from me.

As soon as he injected the iodine into my hand through the catheter IV, I felt extreme, intense pain in my right hand!

I immediately cried out, "Something is very wrong! My hand where the IV is located is hurting very badly! Stop the machine! Come help!"

The technician immediately stopped the CT machine from operating, and came rushing to my right side as the table I was lying on rolled back out of the CT machine.

"Take it off, take it off!" I shouted. "It's killing my hand!"

The technician quickly removed the catheter IV from the top of my right hand.

"Call Dr. Wank," I demanded, "Tell him something has gone terribly wrong!"

A number of CT staff came rushing over and surrounded me while I was still lying on the CT table. They were obviously alarmed but no one said what was wrong.

"Quick, get a heat pack and put it on his hand," someone ordered.

"No ... not heat ... ice is needed," someone else argued.

While the CT staff were debating what should be done, I looked at my right hand and was shocked to see that it had ballooned up grotesquely to nearly double its normal size! Instinctively, I raised my right hand up in the air as high as I could in the hope that so doing might relieve the throbbing, excruciating pain I was feeling.

It didn't help.

Dr. Wank soon arrived and stood at my right side while I was still lying on the CT table. Surrounded by a number of CT staff gathered there, the doctor discovered what went wrong.

"You'll be all right, Mr. Walsh," he assured me. "When the iodine contrast was released, the power of its thrust blew the IV out of the vein in your hand, and forced some of the iodine contrast under the skin of your hand. The swelling you see is from the iodine contrast that was released and trapped under the skin."

Turning to the CT staff, Dr. Wank demanded to know who put the IV in my hand.

When no one answered, I told him, "The IV was put into my hand by someone in that special department where all the phlebotomists are located."

The doctor shook his head, and admonished the CT staff, "All of YOU should know that you **NEVER** put an IV catheter in a patient's hand for a CT scan! It should always be put in the forearm. Otherwise, the power of the thrust of iodine being released can blow the IV right out of the patient's vein ... as happened here!"

I asked, "Doctor, why don't you have the IV put in my forearm **NOW** so the CAT scan can be done so we can see what the cancer is doing inside me."

Dr. Wank replied, "I appreciate your concern, Mr. Walsh. I realize you're anxious to have the CAT scan done so we can learn as much as possible about your condition. However ... you cannot have more iodine injected into your system right now because of what has happened. To put more iodine into your system at this time would be dangerous. It would be too much for your body to safely process."

When I asked him to explain why, he appeared annoyed as if I was asking him to explain something that was abundantly obvious.

Dispute his apparent annoyance, he patiently explained with dramatic emphasis, "Mr. Walsh ... putting more iodine in your body right now would risk doing serious damage to your kidneys and other organs possibly destroying their ability to function properly. Too much iodine could even be fatal!"

After allowing his dramatic words to sink into my now incredulous mind, the doctor added. "You cannot put too much iodine into your system in a short period of time without possibly damaging your kidneys so badly you might have to go on dialysis for the rest of your life! Now, Mr. Walsh ... do you understand why I don't want you to be given any more iodine for the remainder of your stay here at NIH?"

"Yes, of course, I understand, doctor," I replied. "I didn't realize how dangerous it could be to get too much iodine. Thank you for explaining."

Turning to the CT staff still standing nearby, Dr. Wank snapped, "I am putting instructions on this patient's records **that he is not to be given any more iodine for the remainder of his time here this week! Does everyone here understand that?"**

As Dr. Wank stormed off, I found myself still lying on the table partly in the CT machine. I was so stunned by what happened ... and my right hand hurt terribly.

Someone who I assumed was a supervisor in the CT area stayed with me to make sure I was okay ... and that my grotesquely ballooned right hand didn't become worse. Once she was confident I appeared to be okay, she told me I could go back to my hospital room.

"Let the nurse on your floor know what happened," she instructed.

MY JOURNEY WITH NEUROENDOCRINE CANCER
What You Don't Know Can Kill You!

I was then permitted to walk back to my room on the fifth floor in the hospital ... all alone. It occurred to me afterward that NIH procedures needed to be modified for incidents like these. Improvements should include a clear stipulation that any patient who experiences a similar mishap should **NEVER** be allowed to walk back alone to his/her room within the vast NIH complex! Later, after speaking with NIH management, I was assured this procedural improvement was going to be implemented.

I certainly hope so.

As I completed the 10-15 minute walk, I felt light-headed, weak ... and worried. When I got back to my room, my sister, Diana, came by and was shocked to see how badly swollen my right hand looked. She was even more surprised to hear what happened in the CT area causing the injury ... including that I was allowed to walk back to my hospital room unescorted by NIH staff. Diana took a picture of my badly swollen hand.

Two days later on Thursday, November 16, 2017, Dr. Wank decided to have another CT scan done of my abdomen – only this time, he said that it was to be done without the use of iodine contrast for obvious reasons. He said a watery fluid would be used in place of the iodine-based contrast usually used. He explained this would allow imaging of my upper abdomen only, but this would be useful in terms of his team's study of the familial neuroendocrine cancer I had.

As planned, on late Thursday afternoon, the nurse assigned to my room came in and gave me three large bottles of a contrast marked "Iohexol." At the time, I was sitting with two NIH nutritionists who were providing me with important advice on diet and nutrition.

My nurse interrupted our conversation to literally order me to drink the entire contents of the two Iohexol bottles within twenty minutes! She added that I was to take the third bottle of Iohexol down with me to the CT imaging department where she said I must drink it immediately in the presence of a CT staff member before I was to have the scheduled CT scan done.

I reminded her that Dr. Wank was emphatic I should **NOT** be given any more iodine for the remainder of my week at NIH because of the serious mishap that occurred in the CT imaging department two days earlier. I added that Dr. Wank told me that today's scheduled CT scan was to be done **ONLY** with the use of a watery fluid he said was harmless to me. I asked if she was aware of the doctor's instructions he said he was going to enter on my patient records on NIH's system.

She smiled and said she was fully aware of Dr. Wank's instructions and that she had already checked my records on NIH's system. She assured me the Iohexol liquid was okay for me to take for the scheduled CT scan … and that I was to begin drinking the two Iohexol bottles while she stood there, watched me and timed it!

The two nutritionists sitting with me joked about how fortunate I was to drink such a good-tasting, delicious liquid. I drank the Iohexol fluids as quickly as I could. The nurse then told me to "get going" down to the CT area. I excused myself from the two nutritionists and the nurse, and began the long walk down to the CT imaging department on the first floor for the CT scan of my abdomen - the one that was supposed to be done without iodine contrast.

From the moment I arrived in the CT imaging department, I told each CT staff member that my doctor, Dr. Wank, had given very important, emphatic instructions that I was **NOT** to be given any iodine contrast for the CT scan.

When I eventually met the CT technician who was to conduct the CT scan of my abdomen, I told him, "Dr. Wank has ordered that the CT scan I am to get today should only be done with a watery fluid – it is **NOT** to be done with any iodine contrast. He said this is very important, and that his instructions are on my patient records."

Like other NIH staff members I spoke with in the CT area, he assured me that he knew what was required. However, I had the distinct, uneasy impression that no one in the CT area was really listening to anything I said. I wondered if I was just being overly nervous because of the mishap that happened two days before in this same CT department.

I told the CT technician how I had already quickly drunk two bottles of Iohexol when I was up in my hospital room immediately before I came down to the CT imaging department.

Motioning to the third bottle of Iohexol I had in my hand, I asked, "Are you sure, this is safe for me to drink now?"

The technician chuckled and assured me, "Yes, it's safe. We use it all the time. You'll be fine ... please drink it."

I quickly drank the entire contents of the bottle but his words and nonchalant attitude only added to the uneasy impression I had that no one in the CT department was really listening to what I had to say.

"It's late in the day," I thought, "perhaps everyone here has been listening to me but are just hurrying to get the day over with."

I was dead wrong.

While I was lying on the table inside the CT machine, the technician came over to my left side and injected a cool-feeling substance into the IV catheter located in the middle of my left forearm.

As he did, he said, **"Okay, now here comes the iodine,** lay as still as you can while the scan is being done!"

I thought he was kidding when he said, "here comes the iodine!" He can't be serious after all I told him, I thought. When the scan was finished, I asked him if he was kidding when he said, "Here comes the iodine!"

"Did you really inject me with iodine contrast through the IV in my forearm?" I asked.

Incredulously, he answered, "Yes, of course, I did! I used iodine contrast; that's what we always use!"

"Didn't you listen to anything I said?" I shouted.

"What are you talking about," he asked looking concerned. NOW he was finally listening to me! I couldn't believe it! He wasn't kidding!

"Oh, my God," I thought. "He didn't listen to anything I said about Doctor Wank's instructions that I was NOT to be given any more iodine!"

He had actually injected me with more iodine contrast!

"That's standard procedure for this type of CT scan," he nervously explained.

I angrily reminded him how I had repeatedly told him and others in the CT department that Dr. Wank's instructions on NIH's system clearly ordered that I should **NOT** be given any more iodine contrast!

"My God, what's the matter with all you people!" I shouted. "Doesn't anyone here pay attention to the doctor's instructions? You just overdosed me with too much iodine!"

As I said this, I could feel my face and head becoming more and more warm and flushed. Soon, I felt like I was burning up, and the area in the front-bottom area of my neck around my thyroid was aching badly.

Some of the staff in the CT area stopped what they were doing and just stared at me. NOW they were listening! Unbelievable! NOW everyone apparently remembered how I made a big deal earlier about **NOT** being given **ANY** iodine for the CT scan. Despite realizing something had gone terribly wrong, no one called Dr. Wank to tell him what happened to me, his patient.

MY JOURNEY WITH NEUROENDOCRINE CANCER
What You Don't Know Can Kill You!

Then, for the second time in two days, I was allowed to walk unescorted from the CT department on the first floor all the way up to my room on the fifth floor of NIH's hospital. As I did, the deep ache in my thyroid throbbed painfully while my face and head felt red-hot. It was then that a piercing headache started, and I began to feel nauseous.

As soon as I got back to my room on the fifth floor, I told my nurse and my sister, Diana, what happened. My nurse actually appeared to take my words lightly until she went over to NIH's roll-about computer and checked my records. As she read, her expression quickly changed as she realized something went terribly wrong. Without saying a word, she rushed out of my hospital room.

Besides worrying about surviving NET cancer, I then had to worry about what harm was done to me by NIH staff by giving me more iodine than Dr. Wank said was safe. Little did I know at that time but there was more disappointment to come my way at NIH.

Late that night around two in the morning, I felt so sick with a headache, nausea and an ongoing, painful, throbbing ache around my thyroid. When I felt like my throat was beginning to close, I alerted my sister, Diana, and asked her to escort me to the nurse's station on our floor. There, I told the nurse on duty how badly I was suffering, and asked her to please call whomever the doctor was on call at the hospital.

Incredulously, the nurse refused to call the doctor on duty!

"You look just fine to me," she audaciously said. "You are obviously okay! You can wait until morning when a doctor will be available."

I disagreed and strongly reiterated that I needed a doctor to come help me, "I am NOT well. There is something seriously wrong. I feel like my throat is closing. Please call a doctor to come right now!"

Amazingly, this nurse refused to call a doctor! My sister and I could not believe her unprofessional behavior ... and she was the only nurse on the entire floor!

Despite my repeated pleas and insistence, she adamantly refused saying, "I can see you don't need a doctor! You are obviously okay!"

I complained, "You are **NOT** a doctor; you are **NOT** qualified to determine how serious my condition is! Something is seriously wrong! You have no right to refuse to call a doctor!"

I thought, "Oh my God, here I am in the middle of the night far away from home in NIH's hospital in Maryland with my throat closing because NIH's CT staff gave me too much iodine ... and this night nurse won't call the doctor on duty for me!"

My sister and I could not believe it was happening. When I told the night nurse that I was going to call 911 if she did not call a doctor right away, she finally, reluctantly, agreed to call a doctor.

A short time later, one of the doctors on Dr. Wank's team, Dr. Da, spoke to me by telephone. I described how I was erroneously given too much iodine earlier in the CT department, and how my throat hurt and felt like it was closing. After asking several questions, Dr. Da said he didn't think I was in any immediate medical danger.

He spoke to the nurse and instructed her to give me some throat lozenges to relieve the throbbing pain and soreness I felt in my throat. The lozenges helped to relieve some of the intense pain in my throat but I still felt very sick and could not sleep the rest of the night. For the remainder of the night, I worried about what harm had been done to me through NIH's overdose of iodine.

The next morning Dr. Da came by and examined my throat. With my sister, Diana, at my side, the doctor apologized on behalf of NIH for the "mishaps" as he called them. To our surprise, he told us that he had already spoken to staff in the CT department and they admitted what was done wrong!

Shaking his head, Dr. Da stated, "They admitted they inadvertently gave you more iodine. They remember you telling everyone how Dr. Wank said you were not to be given any more iodine. Unfortunately, they did because CT scans are usually done with iodine. They admitted no one checked the system to review Dr. Wank's instructions for you. I checked the system myself earlier and did see that Dr. Wank's instructions were there all the time! Quite apparently, no one in the CT department checked the system before giving you more iodine."

Diana then asked, "Doctor, I find it very disturbing that my brother, a cancer patient here in NIH's hospital, felt he was having a serious medical crisis in the middle of the night but the night nurse refused to call a doctor for him!"

The doctor agreed that should not have happened. "I am surprised and disappointed that the night nurse refused to call a doctor. Her decision not to contact a doctor as requested simply was not appropriate ... especially under those circumstances. No nurse should ever refuse to call a doctor when a patient feels he or she needs one."

Before leaving, the doctor advised me to follow up with my primary care doctor "as soon as you return home."

"You need to have your thyroid and kidneys thoroughly checked to make sure the excess iodine you received didn't cause some harm."

As soon as I got back home on November 18, 2017, I was examined by my primary care physician, Dr. Howard Hertz, in his Babylon, New York office. My throat still hurt badly and I continued to feel quite ill from the overdose of iodine. The doctor had several vials of blood drawn for tests to determine if my thyroid and kidneys were functioning properly. He also prescribed a sonogram be done of my thyroid.

The sonogram was done at Zwanger-Pesiri, Deer Park, New York. Dr. Hertz later told me the results of the sonogram - and the blood tests – indicated my thyroid and kidneys appeared to be okay.

"However," he cautioned, "You won't know for sure if everything is alright until a few months from now when damage to your thyroid ... and/or your kidneys ... might show up."

Before he ended the consult, he asked, "How much iodine did they tell you they actually gave you?"

"They never told me! I've made several requests to NIH but nobody to date has told me just how much excess iodine they gave me. I still don't know."

Dr. Hertz simply shook his head.

MY JOURNEY WITH NEUROENDOCRINE CANCER
What You Don't Know Can Kill You!

Chapter 23

DOCTOR GROSSLY INEPT CRIPPLES ME!

In November 2017, I went to see Dr. Grossly Inept at his "cancer center" on Long Island for my monthly Sandostatin 30 mg injection.

I asked if the monthly Sandostatin injections were intended to treat the area of my ampulla of vater where the original tumor was located, or was it for the lesion on my diaphragm. Dr. Grossly Inept said the Sandostatin treatments were more to prevent the lesion on my ampulla of vater area from returning than they were to prevent the lesion in the left crus of my diaphragm from growing.

The doctor then proceeded to wickedly jam the three-inch needle with Sandostatin (30 mg) into my left buttock muscle. This time, however, unlike previous injections when Dr. Grossly Inept stabbed me with the three-inch needle directly into my buttock muscle, a stabbing, agonizing pain shot all the way down my left leg from the site of the injection to the very tips of my toes!

I realized right away that something very, very bad had just happened. An excruciating pain began to throb from the injection site in my left buttock all the way down my left leg.

Throughout the remainder of the day well into the evening, I suffered unspeakable agony. Around midnight, the pain was so bad, I couldn't walk. I found myself crawling on the floor ... moaning and begging God to please ease the pain. There was no position I could arrange to eased the unrelenting, excruciating pain.

At one point, I decided to go upstairs to my bedroom on the second floor to try to find some relief on my comfortable bed. To reach my bedroom, I crawled to the bottom of the stairs and looked up at the 13 daunting steps I would have to climb. These steps looked so intimidating to me ... like a high, dangerous mountain.

With the lure of possibly getting some relief, however, I

decided to brave the stairs. The only way I could do it, though, was to crawl up the stairs ... head first on my belly one slow, agonizing step at a time. Each step set off excruciating spasms forcing me to freeze where I was until the spasms stopped. It seemed like an eternity, but I finally reached the top of the stairs.

After resting for a while, I struggled to reach up and turn the door knob I had so easily turned so many times in the past. This made me think of so many other things I do that I have taken for granted. As I thought this, I lamented how I have become so incapacitated and tortured by neuroendocrine cancer ... and that damned three-inch needle!

I quickly reminded myself that I must resist such useless, self-pitying thoughts. Slowly crawling, I made my way into the darkened, cool bedroom until I reached my bed. Struggling mightily, I pulled myself up into a kneeling position but could not move further. The pain was just too much to even breathe deeply.

At three o'clock in the morning, I was still kneeling there praying that God would have mercy on me and ease my suffering. This caused me to think of how Jesus suffered so terribly as He knelt in the Garden of Gethsemane. Jesus hurt so badly, He asked God the Father to take away the cup of suffering. But ultimately, Jesus prayed that God the Father's will be done ... not His.

Hurting so badly, I followed Jesus's example by asking God the Father to please take away my suffering, "If it is not Your will, Father, then please give me the strength to bear up under it. At least allow me to find a position where I can better endure this pain!"

As soon as I prayed this, a thought came into my mind to put a pillow on the bed in front of me, then lean as far as I could onto it from the kneeling position I was in. Amazingly, this had the immediate effect of easing the agonizing pain I was suffering. Soon, I was mercifully able to escape the nightmarish pain as I slipped off into a deep slumber.

MY JOURNEY WITH NEUROENDOCRINE CANCER
What You Don't Know Can Kill You!

Every day over the ensuing week, I continued to suffer without much relief day and night. The only way I could get around was to continue slowly crawling around on my hands and knees. Life in general - not just my physical surroundings - created was an entirely different, humbling experience for me. I took nothing for granted ... and respected everyone ... and everything ... as precious gifts from God.

In December, I had been able to resume a little walking - although unsteady at best. Just when it appeared my terribly debilitating condition might be improving, my left leg literally "gave out" at home causing me to take a nasty, painful fall right in front of several family members.

I was in so much pain, I couldn't get up. Family members rushed over to help lift me up off the floor. Besides humiliating me, this fall added to the physical pain I was suffering. It was all so very, very depressing. My injury was so severe, I required the use of a wheelchair to get around anywhere. I once again found myself debilitated and grounded with terrible pain ... as I battled the demons of self-pity.

Being so incapacitated, reminded me of how badly my mother suffered years ago with breast cancer that had metastasized. The cancer caused her great sufferings, torturing her for years but through it all, she never gave up and waged a fierce battle for life until it finally overtook her.

I admired her steadfast bravery and faith. Often, she would tell me that it was helpful to think of others who suffer in worse ways than we do. Like Jesus in the Garden of Gethsemane. Remembering her advice helped me deal with this latest painful time in my life.

I thought back to one time in the middle of the night when my father called and asked me to please come join him in the emergency room where Mom was brought. She was brought there because unbearable pain she was suffering from back pains caused by the cancer.

I remember arriving at the hospital and seeing my Dad in the waiting room sobbing uncontrollably. When he composed himself, he asked me to go into the room where my mother was waiting for some medical help.

"Please go and do something to help Mom," Daddy pleaded. "The doctors have said there is nothing more they can do for her because she has already had far too many powerful pain killers. If they give her any more, they say it will kill her!"

As I approached the room Mom was in, I could hear her crying out in pain. When I entered and went over to her bedside, I wrapped my arms around her as she pleaded with me to do something to ease her pain. All I could do was cry out to God begging Him to help in some way. That moment was one of the saddest, most painful my life. Here was my mother who had given me life, nurtured me and helped me in so many ways throughout my life ... and now she needed me to comfort and help her. I felt so helpless; there was nothing I could do for her but beg God for help.

"Please, God, send somebody to help Mom!"

As soon as I said these words, the door opened and a tall, handsome doctor dressed in brilliant white clothing came in. His appearance was absolutely dazzling in the dimly lit room ... and his countenance brought an immediate sense of peace.

"You called for help ... so here I am!"

"I didn't call out loud, doctor ... but I am happy you are here. My mother desperately needs help; she is suffering terribly from the cancer she has. The other doctors say they can't give her any more pain killers but somebody has to do something to help her."

"Since you called, there **IS** something I can do," he said as he quietly moved over to Mom's bedside. As soon as he arrived there, she gazed up into his eyes and stopped her pitiful screams for help. As I watched, he gently placed his hands on her arms and began softly singing something in barely audible sounds.

Rather than giving Mom some pain killers, this angelic person eased her pain and comforted her through his mere presence and prayerful words. I realized God heard and answered my call for help by sending an angel to comfort Mom.

Remembering this remarkable encounter so many years later, encouraged me to call out to God in my physical agony to ask Him if He could send that angel down to help me now. Well, no one in dazzling white clothing appeared … but the terrible pain I was experiencing quickly vanished.

BOB WALSH

Chapter 24

"DOCTOR PAIN"

In mid-December, I was in so much pain, I went to see a pain management specialist, Dr. Daniel Kohane, in his Bay Shore, Long Island, New York office. My wife, Margie, jokingly calls him "Doctor Pain" because the injections he administers are so painful. Dr. Kohane is a gifted, wonderful doctor who had treated both Margie and me for various back issues over several years.

The doctor read a recent MRI report of my spine, examined me, and then recommended I have an injection of a steroid directly into the lumbar area of my spine. To do so, however, he required that I get medical clearance from my oncologist, Dr. Grossly Inept, and Dr. Howard Hertz, my primary care physician. I faxed the necessary medical clearance forms to be completed over to Dr. Grossly Inept's office along with a copy of the recent MRI radiology report on the lumbar area of my spine.

Although I called and carefully explained the terrible suffering I was in and the need for medical clearance so I could get a pain relief injection, neither Dr. Grossly Inept nor anyone else in his office ever processed the medical clearance form from Dr. Kohane. As a result, Dr. Kohane was forced to cancel the appointment scheduled to provide me with an injection to relieve the terrible pain I was suffering. Every day, I suffered constant, agonizing pain, numbness and tingling in my lower spine and down my left leg. At night, I could not sleep.

Eventually Dr. Kohane was able to administer what are called "trigger shots," pain-relief injections that did not require medical clearance.

In late December, I called Dr. Grossly Inept and told him what happened to me as a result of the last injection he had given me. His only response was to tell me that in all his years he had never had a similar incident with any of his other cancer patients. He was more worried about being sued than he was doing something to help me with the agonizing pain I was suffering from the injection he gave me!

Dr. Grossly Inept never called back to find out how I was doing. For the remainder of December and most of January, I was not able to walk without use of a walker and, at times, a wheelchair, to get around. During the preceding three months, I had fallen so many times I lost count.

I thank God, however because I did not break any bones.

Chapter 25

THE DREADED THREE INCH NEEDLE

As January 2018 began, I was still suffering badly - day and night - from the injury caused by Dr. Grossly Inept when he used the three-inch Sandostatin needle to stab me directly into my left buttock's cheek two months prior.

Seeking relief from the terrible pain - and to understand what was causing such agony - I was very fortunate to get an appointment to see a renowned neuroendocrine cancer oncologist, Dr. Edward M. Wolin, on January 2, 2018.

At the time, Dr. Wolin was located in Montefiore Einstein Center for Cancer Care in Bronx, New York. Dr. Wolin was later appointed Director of "The Center for Carcinoid and Neuroendocrine Tumors" at the Tisch Cancer Institute in Mount Sinai Hospital located in New York City.

After thoroughly reviewing my medical history regarding neuroendocrine cancer, and listening to what Dr. Grossly Inept had been treating me for, Dr. Wolin explained, "The serious pain and debilitation you are suffering was a result of Dr. Grossly Inept injecting you with the three-inch Sandostatin needle directly into your left buttock muscle!

"He should know the three-inch Sandostatin needle should **"NEVER"** be injected straight into the buttock muscle because that is where the sciatic nerve network is located right under the skin!"

For emphasis, he stated**, "The Sandostatin needle should always be injected into the buttock muscle from the side ... not directly in from the front!"**

"That is what crippled you ... not the cancer!"

There are no words to adequately describe how greatly disturbed I felt to learn the terrible, agonizing pain I suffered for many months was because Dr. Grossly Inept improperly injected me with the three-inch needle.

I vented incredulously, "I cannot believe this! Dr. Grossly Inept crippled me with a three-inch needle because he didn't know how to properly administer it! How can he present himself to cancer patients as being an experienced, qualified NET oncologist, and yet not know how to properly administer the three-inch Sandostatin needle?

"And what about the pharmaceutical company that manufactures Sandostatin ... Novartis Pharmaceutical? Shouldn't Novartis as the manufacturer of Sandostatin and the related three-inch needle be required by the FDA to advise oncologists on the proper way Sandostatin should be used when injecting NET cancer patients with it?"

(Novartis Pharmaceutical is the U.S. arm of Novartis International AG, a Swiss multinational pharmaceutical company that is based in Basel, Switzerland.)

I wanted to find out if Novartis Pharmaceutical maintained appropriate policies and procedures that ensured all oncologists who used their Sandostatin product knew how to properly administer it to NET cancer patients. Shockingly, all my attempts to contact someone, anyone, at Novartis Pharmaceutical were unsuccessful.

It became painfully apparent that Novartis Pharmaceutical was allowed by U.S. laws to dispense Sandostatin to NET cancer patients without any consequence when something goes so terribly wrong to the cancer patient using their product as happened in my case.

It also became painfully obvious that Novartis does not care enough for NET cancer patients - their ultimate customers - because Novartis doesn't provide some form of communications with NET cancer patients who use their Sandostatin product.

To add insult to injury, I discovered something else that

MY JOURNEY WITH NEUROENDOCRINE CANCER
What You Don't Know Can Kill You!

Novartis does that absolutely infuriated me. I learned that Dr. Grossly Inept and other oncologists are actually rewarded by Novartis Pharmaceutical when the doctors administer Sandostatin rather than other medications to treat NET cancer!

All this left me feeling obligated to issue a warning to other NET cancer patients. When it comes to neuroendocrine cancer treatments, be careful when dealing with Novartis and Sandostatin!

I realized I had to find a different oncologist who could properly administer the monthly Sandostatin three-inch needle injections. I couldn't ask Dr. Wolin to administer the injections because he was due to go to Mount Sinai Hospital in New York City and would not be settled for a few months.

I asked Dr. Wolin if he knew of another oncologist on Long Island to whom he could refer for further neuroendocrine cancer treatments until he got to Mount Sinai Hospital. He couldn't recommend anyone at the time, and so, I was forced to continue seeing Dr. Grossly Inept for a while longer.

"God help me," I thought.

BOB WALSH

MY JOURNEY WITH NEUROENDOCRINE CANCER
What You Don't Know Can Kill You!

Chapter 26

BLOOD TESTS ALONE CAN MISS NET CANCER!

With no other choice at the time, on January 8, 2018, I went to an appointment with Dr. Grossly Inept. I told him what Dr. Wolin said about the proper way of injecting the three-inch Sandostatin needle. Dr. Grossly Inept appeared impressed to hear this ... and said that is how he would administer the Sandostatin needle from then on.

The doctor, looking embarrassed, said nothing else as he quickly went about administering the three-inch needle. Afterward, I once again suffered for 10 to 14 days with flu-like symptoms.

A few weeks later, on February 5, 2018, my wife, Margie, and my sister, Diana, joined me for another appointment with Dr. Grossly Inept. During our visit, Dr. Grossly Inept appeared to be trying to impress Diana as he bragged about having "extensive experience and knowledge of neuroendocrine cancer."

At one point, Diana asked him the significance of the special blood tests that are run to assess the presence of neuroendocrine cancer in the body.

Dr. Grossly Inept stood as if he was a professor delivering a lecture in front of a class as he boasted, "I can tell you definitively ... from my experience ... if the 'special' blood tests come back negative, then that patient does NOT have neuroendocrine cancer!"

Diana laughed loudly and boldly corrected him, "Doctor, what you are saying is absolutely not correct! And you should NOT be giving that terrible misinformation to patients!"

Dr. Grossly Inept was clearly stunned to silence by Diana's aggressive words and demeanor.

"Let me explain something to you, Doctor," Diana continued. "Last year, I had all those 'special' blood tests done and they came back perfectly normal. Rather than accept those words as being correct, I had a colonoscopy done a week later. **The colonoscopy clearly showed I had five malignant neuroendocrine tumors in my ileum!**

"If I had listened to doctors like you, this deadly cancer would have spread before I had any chance of fighting it!

"Just to be sure you get what I am telling you, doctor … listen to me! There is no way that … 'special blood tests' … are sufficient alone to detect the presence of neuroendocrine cancer! There are other diagnostic tests that must be done!"

I couldn't tell if Dr. Grossly Inept was more annoyed or embarrassed as he quickly darted from the room without saying another word. He returned moments later with the three-inch Sandostatin needle and gruffly administered it - into the side of my buttock muscle.

Afterward, he handed me a completed medical clearance form for Dr. Kohane so I could get the pain-relief injection in my spine for the pain I was still suffering from the November 2017 Sandostatin injection Dr. Grossly Inept had given me. Everyone then vacated the room without a single other word being spoken.

Once again, for the entire following week, I felt as if I had a wicked case of the flu including headache, nausea, lethargy and stool that was consistently light tan in color.

And yes … I still had occasional facial flushing as well.

Chapter 27

"YOU MAY NEVER FULLY HEAL!"

On February 14, 2018, I went to see Dr. Alan Mechanic, a highly regarded neurosurgeon, at his Commack, New York office. This consult was arranged to get the doctor's advice about the injury to the sciatic nerves in my spine, and the related injury to my left knee from a subsequent fall.

After reviewing the medical records I provided, the doctor examined me then told me the injury to my sciatic nerves in my spine from the Sandostatin injection appeared to be slowly healing.

"However," he added, "It might take a full year or more before everything fully recovers. It is also quite possible the injury to your sciatic nerves may never fully heal."

God help me.

BOB WALSH

Chapter 28

DOCTOR PAIN TRIES TO HELP

On February 16, 2018, I gave Dr. Daniel Kohane(whom my wife Margie has kiddingly nicknamed "Dr. Pain"), Pain Management Physician, the medical clearance forms from Dr. Hertz and Dr. Grossly Inept so he could schedule a steroid injection in the lumbar area of my spine. In terms of the left knee injury, he said the MRI showed the injury was a torn meniscus.

Since I was still suffering non-stop, agonizing pain day and night from the injury to my sciatic nerve from the November 2017 Sandostatin injection, on February 19, 2018, Dr. Daniel Kohane injected a pain-relief steroid directly into the lumbar area of my spine. This brought a little, temporary relief to the intense pain I had been suffering … but not the neuropathy which relentlessly continued.

On April 9, 2018, I was still suffering badly from the injury to my sciatic nerve from the November 2017 Sandostatin injection Dr. Grossly Inept incorrectly administered directly into my buttock muscle (rather than from the side of the muscle).

To seek some relief, a steroid injection was administered into the left and right side of the lumbar area of my spine by Dr. Daniel Kohane, pain management physician. The procedure was done in his medical office on Saxon Avenue in Bay Shore, NY. The injections were very painful but over subsequent weeks, I gradually began to feel more mobile. Unfortunately, the torturous neuropathy pain continued created.

BOB WALSH

Chapter 29

NEEDLE BIOPSY OF MY THYROID

On March 29, 2018, Dr. Arnbjorn Toset, a doctor specializing in thyroid, head and neck surgery, came to my primary care physician's office, Dr. Howard Hertz, on Main Street in Babylon, New York. There, Dr. Toset performed a needle biopsy on the left side of my thyroid where there is an enlarged nodule. The procedure, done without anesthesia, was very, very painful as the doctor dug around my thyroid to retrieve several biopsies needed.

As I suffered terribly, I begged God to help me with the excruciating pain. Unfortunately, the level of mind-bending pain remained the same ... but my ability to endure it increased as I thought about how other cancer patients also suffer as they endure different procedures required to diagnose, monitor and treat the cancers they have.

The thought came to mind, "Why waste all this terrible suffering?"

I offered up my sufferings to God for the benefit of the holy souls in Purgatory. Thank God, soon after I said this prayer, the doctor stopped the torturous digging around in my throat. He was finally able to retrieve the number of biopsy specimens needed. What a relief! But then came the long, worrisome, nerve-racking wait for the pathology results to learn whether or not the neuroendocrine cancer in my abdomen and near my spine had metastasized to my thyroid - or if the iodine overdose at NIH had done any damage.

Such waiting, wondering and worrying is yet another sinister way we cancer patients suffer. There are so many times like these that we find ourselves waiting and waiting - to hear some news, any news - about the deadly cancer growing inside our bodies. Despite my repeated calls to Dr. Hertz and Dr. Toset's offices, I wasn't able to get results of the needle biopsies of my thyroid from the staff of either doctor.

Other NET cancer patients have told me how they have suffered in similar ways involving the professional failure by their doctors and staff to communicate critical lab results. It is quite apparent that staff employed by many doctors today are not properly trained - or supervised. One doctor told me a number of practices today employ a central administrative group to handle clerical and administrative duties. What results is little or no accountability for clerical staff who cause patients to suffer the consequences. Even patients with incurable cancer like me.

It wasn't until May 15, 2018 that I was finally able to get an office manager at Dr. Hertz's office to check into - and locate - the pathology report on my thyroid biopsies. Unbelievably, she said the report was dated April 1, 2018 but she said Dr. Hertz's office did not receive the report until April 17, 2018.

I said, "I cannot believe you just said that! Your office got that report on April 17th but today is May 15th - 28 days later - but I had that procedure in your office seven week ago! Seven weeks ago! The only way I found out the report was available was through repeated calls begging for an update! Why in God's name didn't someone in your office call me with critical report that we now know was sitting in your office for four weeks?"

Sounding quite annoyed, her terse reply was, "I don't know, Mr. Walsh. Things can sometimes fall between the cracks ... especially when things can get terribly busy here. Is there anything else I can help you with?"

"Yes. Please tell me if the pathology report I have been so desperately calling for over seven weeks states whether or not the neuroendocrine cancer I have has spread to my thyroid."

She matter-of-factly replied, "No, it doesn't."

MY JOURNEY WITH NEUROENDOCRINE CANCER
What You Don't Know Can Kill You!

I was so greatly relieved to hear this good news but I remained very upset and disappointed at how poorly all of this was handled by Dr. Hertz' staff. I couldn't believe that such a critical report actually sat in the doctor's office for 28 long, long days while I agonized to know if the neuroendocrine cancer had spread to my thyroid. How sad, how very, very sad it is that people can be so uncaring and unprofessional.

I ended our conversation by saying, "I need a copy of that report. Would you please put a copy on your front desk so I can come by and pick it up. (The policy in the doctor's office is that they will not mail copies of lab results to patients. If a patient wants a copy, he must call ahead and request a copy be placed on the front desk for him to pick up.)

Once before when I was feeling desperately ill, I asked if they would make an exception to their policy and mail a copy of a lab report to me. I explained that I was fighting a painful form of incurable cancer and travelling to their office only to get a copy of my lab results was a great difficulty. The blunt, dispassionate answer was, "there are no exceptions.)

I know that Dr. Henry Hertz is a very good doctor and quite compassionate but how this experience was handled by his staff is a mystery to me. Having said that, it is highly likely the doctor has no idea how poorly his staff treated me ... perhaps others.

Having experienced so many similar misdeeds in many other walks of life in our society today, I have come to call such outrageous behavior, **"America today!"**

BOB WALSH

MY JOURNEY WITH NEUROENDOCRINE CANCER
What You Don't Know Can Kill You!

Chapter 30

A SECOND KILLER TUMOR APPEARS!

On July 25, 2018, a sharp, excruciating pain radiated across the center of my digestive system like a bolt of lightning doubling me over. "God help me; here we go again," I lamented. This sudden, unexplained physical pain ebbed and flowed throughout the night until the early morning hours of the next day.

Fortunately, I was able to get an appointment with my primary care physician, Dr. Howard Hertz. After examining me, the doctor ordered a number of tests including a MRI with MRCP of my abdomen to determine the source of my pain. He was concerned as I was that the neuroendocrine cancer was the cause of my suffering.

The very next day, a MRI with MRCP was done at Zwanger-Pesiri in Deer Park, Long Island. The radiologist who reviewed the MRI compared it to the MRI that had been done a year earlier on February 10, 2017.

His report stated, in part, **"the common bile duct still abruptly tapers at the ampulla but no discrete ampullary mass is appreciated."**

I thought his report required additional information so I called the radiologist and asked him to state in an amended report exactly how "abruptly narrowed my common bile duct was at the ampulla." It seemed only obvious to me that oncologists treating me would need a relative number to gauge the seriousness of the narrowing.

I also asked why he failed to recommend that I follow up with my doctors regarding the abrupt narrowing at my ampulla especially since he knew I was already diagnosed with ampulla cancer at that specific site.

His answer surprised me, "We simply disagree, Mr. Walsh. I do not think it is necessary to recommend any follow up!"

"Why?" I asked.

"Because you already know you have neuroendocrine cancer at the ampulla. Besides, I don't see any tumors; I only see an abrupt narrowing!"

After further discussion, this radiologist eventually agreed to provide an amended report that contained a number describing just how narrowed my common bile duct was at the site of my ampulla. He stated my common bile duct was virtually closed but he just couldn't bring himself to write zero. Instead, he listed the opening of the narrowed area as being 1 mm.

His amended radiology report on my patient portal at the Zwanger-Pesiri website stated in an addendum, "The common bile duct narrows approximately 5 mm upstream to the ampulla and measures less than 1 mm in diameter following its abrupt narrowing. No discrete ampullary mass is identified that would correspond to the known neuroendocrine tumor."

Research I conducted on neuroendocrine cancer indicated that such abrupt narrowing in the common bile duct at the ampulla may indicate the presence of an aggressive malignancy.

On August 25, 2018, I made an appointment with a local oncologist for her advice. My wife, Margie, and I visited Dr. Mary Puccio, oncologist, in her Bay Shore, Long Island, New York office. After thoroughly reviewing my medical history including all recent MRI reports, Dr. Puccio prescribed a 68-gallium Dota-tate full body CT/PET scan be conducted as soon as possible to determine what role neuroendocrine cancer may be playing in my common bile duct … and possibly elsewhere.

Accordingly, on August 27, 2018, a 68-gallium Dota-tate scan full body CT/PET scan was done at the Northwell Imaging Center in Bay Shore, New York. Two days later, we met with Dr.

MY JOURNEY WITH NEUROENDOCRINE CANCER
What You Don't Know Can Kill You!

Puccio who told us what radiologists at Northwell Imaging had to report. She began by telling us they compared their findings with those Northwell reported on another CT/PET scan done more than a year earlier on March 27, 2017.

This report stated there was tracer uptake in my common bile duct at the ampulla "consistent with the known neuroendocrine tumor. Alarmingly, the SUV (standard uptake value) of that area was 19.1; the SUV a year earlier was only 14.9. A higher SUV level is known to indicate a highly aggressive malignancy.

As a next step, Dr. Puccio recommended I have an endoscopy with EUS and ERCP of my abdomen ... as soon as it can be arranged. And so, I made an appointment for a consultation with Dr. Raj Bansal, gastroenterologist who was familiar with my medical condition since he twice before conducted an endoscopy with EUS and ERCP a year earlier.

In making this appointment, I explained to his secretary why I needed this consult so that an endoscopy with EUS and ERCP could be done as soon as possible. Despite explaining the circumstances of my present medical condition, his secretary said I would have to wait a few weeks before I could see the doctor!

Those weeks passed very, very slowly for me as I prayed and worried, prayed and worried, prayed and worried, and then prayed and worried some more. Living with a terminal, incurable cancer has a way at times like these of dramatically slowing the passing of time.

Then, unfortunately, a few days before the consult was to take place, his secretary called to tell me the doctor had to cancel the appointment. Under the circumstances, I requested the next earliest appointment for a consult. She shocked me by saying quite matter-of-factly that the next available appointment was several more weeks from then! I implored her under my dire circumstances to please give me an earlier appointment.

"My recent scans clearly show how the malignant neuroendocrine cancer in me is growing and the only way oncologists can determine what steps to take requires that an endoscopy be done as soon as possible."

It was as if she wasn't listening as she said "the best she could" do was to give me an appointment three weeks away! No amount of explaining could influence her to give me an earlier appointment. Under the circumstances, I had no choice but to wait … and pray … wait and pray … wait and pray … wait and pray.

When that second appointment finally approached, Dr. Bansal's secretary called a few days before and once again cancelled the appointment! This second time left me completely stunned and disturbed.

I could only assume Dr. Bansal was not aware his appointments secretary was doing something I felt was simply outrageous. Waiting to see him had cost me two valuable months in my struggle with a rare, incurable, malignancy growing inside me.

As soon as I hung up with Dr. Bansal's secretary, I immediately called for a consultation with Dr. Myron Schwartz, the director of surgery at the Neuroendocrine Cancer Center at Mount Sinai Hospital in New York City. Unlike dealing with Dr. Bansal's staff, Dr. Schwartz' representative patiently and efficiently gathered all pertinent information related to my health issues … and scheduled an appointment for me to see Dr. Schwartz the very next week!

Although Mount Sinai and North Shore Hospital are part of the same Northwell System, it was quite apparent that Dr. Schwartz and Mount Sinai Hospital maintained a much higher standard in handling quality of care issues in support of medical services. This may not seem very important to most people, however, to cancer patients like me dealing with an incurable malignancy it makes a great deal of difference.

MY JOURNEY WITH NEUROENDOCRINE CANCER
What You Don't Know Can Kill You!

Administrative and clerical issues matter. North Shore Hospital would do well to learn how Mount Sinai Hospital is able to maintain such a high quality of care ... and follow their example!

On September 19, 2018, my wife, Margie, and I attended a consultation meeting with Dr. Schwartz and his staff at Mount Sinai hospital in New York City. After thoroughly reviewing my scans, pathology and radiology reports, Dr. Schwartz focused on the recent 68-gallium Dota-tate CT/PET scan of my abdomen. He advised us that he concurred with the radiology findings that indicated there was an ominous area where neuroendocrine cancer was situated in the very bottom of my common bile duct right at the ampulla.

I asked him to explain what the tumor's SUV (standard uptake value) indicated on this recent scan.

"Well," he began with an ominous tone in his voice, "I am afraid the higher SUV on this scan unfortunately indicates the tumor is now much larger - and more aggressive than what was seen on the CT/PET scan last year."

Without further comment on this, he added, "It might be possible for us to do an 'ampullectomy' during an endoscopy to remove the cancerous tissue. This can only be done if the cancer has not spread into the surrounding area.

"In an ampullectomy, the doctor removes the ampulla and as much of the surrounding cancerous area as possible. The remaining area is then closed off by carefully attaching what is left together."

"How effective is this," Margie wanted to know.

"We have found this procedure is quite effective. However, every patient is a unique physical environment therefore specific circumstances always dictate what can be come and affect results. Having said that, I can tell you we have had great experience performing ampullectomies ... and patients typically recover quite well following the procedure.

"To determine whether or not an ampullectomy may be done

in your husband's case, an endoscopy is needed with EUS and ERCP. This can be done here at Mount Sinai if you wish."

I asked Dr. Schwartz how capable and experienced the Mount Sinai doctors were who wound be performing the procedure. I was concerned because I knew the procedure came with some very real, serious risks.

One of Dr. Schwartz' colleagues surprised us by calling out his confident reply, "Mr. Walsh, we do ampullectomies all the time; they are actually quite fun to do!"

Dr. Schwartz added, "Doctor Christopher DiMaio, head of our gastroenterology department, has extensive experience with this procedure and can do the endoscopy here at Mount Sinai if you would like. Would you like me to speak with him and have him call you to make arrangements?"

"Yes, please do," I quickly answered.

Margie and I asked several questions related to this procedure and my particular case of neuroendocrine cancer. The doctor listened carefully and patiently answered our questions and concerns. We left this meeting feeling highly confident we were in the hands of highly capable medical professionals who were thoroughly familiar with neuroendocrine cancer.

I immediately called and made an appointment to have the needed endoscopy done by Dr. DiMaio on October 2, 2018 at Mount Sinai Hospital in upper Manhattan in New York City.

On that day just prior to the procedure, Dr. DiMaio spent considerable time with Margie and me as he thoroughly reviewed my various health issues, and explained the endoscopy procedure.

In particular, he stressed, "The principle purpose of this endoscopy is to identify if the cancer we see on your recent CT/PET scan has spread to the surrounding area. That will help us determine whether or not an ampullectomy may be done at a later date.

MY JOURNEY WITH NEUROENDOCRINE CANCER
What You Don't Know Can Kill You!

"To be sure you understand, Mr. Walsh, I am **NOT** going to do an ampullectomy today ... even if it appears one may be done at this time. I **AM** planning to take several biopsies throughout your system, and I will also take a number of photos.

"When our pathology department reports their findings on the biopsies, I will confer with Doctors Schwartz and Wolin and then share with you our observations and recommendations."

Margie said she hoped the results would be the same as what happened a year earlier. "A malignant tumor in that same area had closed off Bob's entire biliary system leaving him in danger of dying. That is when God intervened and miraculously took the tumor away without surgery or chemo! It was a miracle."

Dr. DiMaio smiled, "Well, from what I read of your husband's medical records, I have to say what happened was really quite amazing. But from what we now see on his recent CT/PET scan, we must deal in science ... not miracles."

With that, he rushed off saying, "I'll come talk with both of you as soon as I complete the procedure today."

Margie and I were left sitting comfortably in a quiet area not far from the operating room. Not knowing what news this day may bring, we did what came so easily. We prayed. We thanked God for all He has done for us and our loved ones ... and we asked Him to pour His healing graces down upon us, the doctors, other patients, all those who suffer and our loved ones. Praying together brought such peace to both of us as I was then led off to the operating room.

Once there, Dr. DiMaio again went over everything pertinent for my benefit, the anesthesiologist and other attending staff. When he finished, the anesthesiologist explained that he was going to inject me with Octreotide which he held up for me to see. The Octreotide was in a bottle no more than one inch long.

"Anyone who has neuroendocrine cancer as you do, must receive this Octreotide before general anesthesia is administered," he elaborated before injecting it in my left shoulder. He then said he was going to administer the general anesthesia. Within a few moments, I felt myself peacefully drift away from consciousness and present time leaving me an utterly peaceful state of being.

When I awoke in recovery, Margie came in and greeted me, "Okay, enough of this sleeping in the middle of the day! The doctor is coming in soon to tell us what he saw."

Just as she finished saying this, Dr. DiMaio, in fact, walked in almost as if on cue.

He looked perplexed as he launched into a report of what he saw. "I did **NOT** see any sign of cancer ... anywhere! I took many biopsies and photos of your esophagus, stomach, common bile duct, ampulla, small intestine, liver, gallbladder and pancreas."

After these wonderful, remarkable words, the doctor fell silent. He literally just stopped talking.

Margie broke the awkward silence by asking a perfectly pointed, frank question, "How can this be, doctor? How can you say there is nothing there when the 68-Gallium CT/PET scan clearly shows there is neuroendocrine tumor with a high SUV uptake indicating it is a highly aggressive malignancy?!"

"I am sorry, Mrs. Walsh, I can't explain it. I am just as mystified as you are," the doctor confessed. "This is not at all what I expected. This just doesn't make any scientific sense! I can only tell you I did not see any sign of the cancerous tumor ... anywhere in your husband's digestive system.

"Mind you, this procedure today did **NOT** plan to include looking at any other place in your husband's body where other oncologists have previously found clinical evidence of at least one other active neuroendocrine tumor near Mr. Walsh's spine.

"I can only assure the both of you that I very carefully, thoroughly looked everywhere in the digestive system and took many, many biopsies. I know I saw it on the recent CT/PET scan but I assure you, but I assure you I did not see any sign of the neuroendocrine tumor in today's procedure. I quite frankly do not understand this."

Margie quickly added, "Well we certainly do! This tumor miraculously disappeared just like the first one did a year ago!"

Dr. DiMaio smiled, "As I mentioned earlier, I am guided by science. Let's wait until the biopsies are reviewed by our pathologists who are well experienced with neuroendocrine cancer. Then, perhaps, we will have a better understanding of what is going on. I will call you at soon as the pathology report is available."

Margie and I went home later that day filled with joy, praise and thanksgiving to God who had quite apparently once again had miraculously interceded to cause a deeply entrenched malignant tumor to literally disappear.

My joy didn't last too long. The very next day, I awoke in horrific pain. I was suffering from what appeared to be pancreatitis, an inflammation of the pancreas. That is one of the possible side effects of having an endoscopy done with EUR and ERCP since that procedure includes obtaining a biopsy from the pancreas. The pain I was experiencing felt like a muscle in my upper, middle torso area was spasmodically twisting.

I went to a local health clinic where a doctor conducted blood tests of my amylase and lipase levels. These hormones are created by pancreas. The doctor explained if these two levels are elevated, this usually indicates pancreatitis. The tests later came back negative. The excruciating pain I suffered lasted five days, and apparently was caused by the many biopsies taken by Dr. DiMaio during the endoscopy with EUS and ERCP.

BOB WALSH

Chapter 31

GOD DOES IT AGAIN - A SECOND MIRACLE!

A week following the special endoscopy at Mount Sinai Hospital in New York City, Dr. Christopher DiMaio called me to convey the results of the biopsies he had taken during the procedure.

"Mr. Walsh ... all the biopsies came back negative! All of them! I do not understand how this can be. Your recent CT/PET scan clearly shows the presence of a significant lesion located in the distal area of your common bile duct. In doing the procedure, however, I did not see anything at all that looked suspicious to me. Now our pathologists have confirmed there was no sign of cancer in any of the biopsies!"

I immediately began to realize that God had just performed a second miracle in removing another deadly NET tumor! Although I have been blessed in my life to witness countless miracles including the disappearance of the first NET tumor a year earlier - I confess this time, I was completely surprised.

While Dr. DiMaio began trying to make sense out of what happened to this second NET tumor, I began to understand why perhaps God did this again. After I told many people how God had miraculously removed the first NET tumor, there really weren't too many people I can say outwardly were impressed. So a year earlier, God performed another, virtually identical, miracle!

I asked the doctor if he could think of any possible scientific explanation for how this tumor simply disappeared.

His emphatic response was, "No, Mr. Walsh; I cannot. I cannot think of a single scientific, medical basis to explain this! In all my years of practice, I have never experienced anything even close to this. This is truly amazing."

I was so elated to hear this but the thought occurred to me,

"Well, what do I so now?"

"You must follow up with Dr. Wolin right away," he advised. "That tumor may have mysteriously disappeared, but the cancer you have has not. It is still in your body."

After a pause, he added, "Doctor Wolin ... like the rest of us ... is now even more anxious for you to continue your care here at Mount Sinai. And now, it is not just because you have the rarest form of the rarest cancer."

Before hanging up, Dr. DiMaio said, "You can tell you wife that I cannot disagree with her any longer. She may be right after all ... what has happened may, in fact, be miraculous."

Thank you, God.

Chapter 32

THE GREATEST MEDICINE OF ALL

Up to this point, I have taken you with me as I looked back on my painful journey with neuroendocrine (NET) cancer. I tried hard not to "sugar-coat" any of the terrible realities of what this rare cancer and others can do to its victims. I also did not pull any punches when it came to sharing some of the outrageous times when a number of doctors and oncologists grossly misinformed me ... and even mistreated me.

Among the many helpful things I learned, there are a few important, fundamental things we cancer patients can do for ourselves.
- First of all ... do get a second and even a third medical opinion (if your insurance coverage allows) for critical health issues such as neuroendocrine cancer.
- Secondly, do NOT accept any doctor or oncologist's verbal opinion that is solely based upon his/her assumption or theory! Insist on having specific, documented scientific evidence to substantiate the doctor or oncologist's diagnosis.
- Lastly, but most important, immerse yourself in prayer and faith! For those of us who are Catholic, remember, the greatest prayer of all is the Holy Sacrifice of the Mass, the Eucharist.

As a Catholic, I discovered this last step contained the secret to true healing and living in peace and happiness in life ... including with the shroud of cancer encasing me. No matter how difficult and truly painful life's journey can be at times, when we turn to God, He helps us carry the burden. I know because He has done so for me countless times. There is no better way to enjoy life's good times, and the painful ones than to allow God's words in holy scripture to guide the way.

All forms of prayer are good, however, I thought it might be helpful to offer a suggested way to pray for healing. Here are the five steps I find most essential:

1. First, you must forgive everyone, everything ... and that includes forgiving yourself which may be the most difficult forgiveness to give. This first step is so important Christ tells us in Matthew 5:25 if we bring gifts to the church but harbor some unforgiveness in our hearts, we should put the gifts down and first go make peace! Note when He tells us to forgive, **He encourages us to forgive as He forgives ... not our way. Several times in the Bible, God tells us when He forgives, He also forgets!**

    In terms of forgiveness, please take a moment to consider what God tells us in the Bible.
    - In St. Paul's letter to the Hebrews 10:17, God says, "Their sins and inequities I will remember no more."
    - In Isaiah 43:18, God says, "Do not remember the former things, or consider the things of old."
    - In Jeremiah 31:34, God says, "I will forgive their iniquity and remember their sin no more."
    - In Isaiah 43:25, God says, "I wipe out your offenses; your sins I will remember no more."

    Clearly, God is telling us to forgive and forget as He does.

2. The next step is for you to clearly tell God what you want

MY JOURNEY WITH NEUROENDOCRINE CANCER
What You Don't Know Can Kill You!

Him to do for you. In Matthew 9:27 Jesus shows us how important this is. He asks two blind men what they want Him to do for them. Note that Jesus does not ask them if they want to see. Jesus certainly knows what we need but He obviously wants us to express faith in Him by actually saying the words. So make sure to ask God for whatever is most important to you ... and don't limit what you ask of Him! While you have the opportunity to ask, consider asking Jesus to help others in your life as well.

3. This next step in healing prayer is also vital - it involves expressing faith in Him once again. Using the example of the two blind men, Jesus tells us how He asks both of them if they believe He can do what they ask of Him ... that is to cure their blindness. When they answered, "Yes, Lord," Jesus replied by saying something quite extraordinary in terms of receiving what we ask of Jesus. He said, "According to your faith, let it be done to you!"

   Remember His words when you pray to Him. Believe with all your heart that Jesus truly can and will do whatever is best for you and for those you pray for. True faith includes understanding that Jesus will always do what is best ... in the very best way ... and very best time.

4. The fourth step involves acknowledging what Jesus does for you by thanking Him. This is so important to Jesus that He gives us a dramatic example in Luke 17:11 when only one leper out of ten healed by Jesus came back to thank Him. Jesus said, "Were not ten cleansed? Where are the other nine lepers?" Jesus is telling us loud and clear it is important to make time to thank God for all He does for us

and for our loved ones. By the way, tradition tells us that Jesus further rewarded the leper by restoring all that he had lost to leprosy! (Leprosy causes the flesh to rot resulting in the loss of fingers, toes, and more body parts.) Then Jesus rewarded the leper in yet the most important way when He said, "Arise, go your way, for your faith has saved you!" Whatever you do, make sure to take time to thank God for what He does for you.

5. For those of us who are Catholics, this final step represents the greatest healing prayer of all in which we unite our prayers for healing with that of the Holy Sacrifice of the Mass, the Eucharist. At every Mass, a miracle takes place when the priest consecrates the bread and wine into the Body and Blood of Our Lord and Savior, Jesus Christ. Following this most sacred of all moments, is one of the greatest healing prayers we can say ... "Lord, I am not worthy that you should come under my roof ... but only say the word ... and my soul shall be healed!"

In closing, I offer this prayer for all readers. May God heal all your wounds, dry every tear, ease your fears and provide what you need for your journey. May you always feel His loving presence ... especially in difficult, trying times. And on some beautiful, glorious day, may He personally welcome you into His loving embrace in Paradise where you will no longer suffer but enjoy everlasting love, peace and happiness. Amen.

SECTION TWO – TECHNICAL REFERENCES

Chapter 33
THE NEUROENDOCRINE SYSTEM

Any discussion regarding neuroendocrine (NET) cancer requires a basic understanding of the neuroendocrine system and what neuroendocrine cells do in the human body.

Neuroendocrine cells receive neuronal input (neurotransmitters[13] released by nerve cells or neurosecretory cells) and, as a consequence of this input, they release message molecules (hormones) to the blood. In that way, they bring about an integration between the nervous system and the endocrine system, a vital process known as "neuroendocrine integration."

An example of a neuroendocrine cell is a cell of the adrenal medulla (the innermost part of the adrenal gland) which releases adrenaline to the blood. Adrenal medullary cells are controlled by the sympathetic division of the autonomic nervous system. These cells are modified postganglionic neurons. Autonomic nerve fibers lead directly to them from the central nervous system.

The adrenal medullary hormones are kept in vesicles much in the same way neurotransmitters are kept in neuronal vesicles. Hormonal effects can last up to ten times longer than those of neurotransmitters. Sympathetic nerve fiber impulses stimulate the release of adrenal medullary hormones. In this way, the

---

[13] **Neurotransmitters** - Also known as chemical messengers, neurotransmitters are endogenous chemicals that enable neurotransmission. They transmit signals across a chemical synapse, such as a neuromuscular junction, from one neuron (nerve cell) to another "target" neuron, muscle cell, or gland cell.

sympathetic division of the autonomic nervous system and the medullary secretions function together.

The major center of neuroendocrine integration in the body is found in the hypothalamus and the pituitary gland. That is where hypothalamic neurosecretory cells release factors to the blood. Some of these factors (releasing hormones), released at the hypothalamic median eminence, control the secretion of pituitary hormones, while others (the hormones oxytocin and vasopressin) are released directly into the blood.

Chapter 34

NEUROENDOCRINE CANCER

Neuroendocrine cancer, often called NET cancer by patients, is a disease of the endocrine system involving abnormal cell growth that forms neuroendocrine tumors (NETs), neoplasms, that arise from cells of the endocrine (hormonal) and nervous systems.

NETs arise from various neuroendocrine cells whose normal function is to serve as the neuroendocrine interface. Neuroendocrine cells are present not only in endocrine glands throughout the body that produce hormones, but also diffusely in all body tissues. It is believed that neuroendocrine cells can de-differentiate into tumor cells.

According to the National Cancer Institute of the National Institutes of Health (NIH), the most common sites where carcinoids tumors (NETs) are found is in the gastrointestinal tract. These tumors are frequently found in the small intestine, stomach and rectum. But because the cells that carcinoid tumors are created from are found throughout the body, these tumors can be found just about anywhere, including the appendix, the colon, the pancreas and the lungs.

Many NETs can be benign but most are malignant with the potential to invade and/or spread to other parts of the body. NETs most commonly occur in the intestine where they are often called carcinoid tumors but they are also found in the pancreas, lung and the rest of the body. There are many kinds of NET tumors. In fact, a NET tumor showed up in a lymph node in my diaphragm while another one showed up in the distal (bottom) area of my common bile duct right at my ampulla of vater effectively closing off my entire biliary system.

Regardless of size, NET tumors can cause considerable harm to the body. Tumors, even if they are very small, can produce adverse effects by secreting hormones. NET tumors are treated as a group of tissue because the cells of these neoplasms share common features including the following:
- they look similar;
- they have special secretory granules; and,
- they often produce biogenic amines and polypeptide hormones.

10% or less of carcinoids, primarily some midgut carcinoids, secrete excessive levels of a range of several type of hormones, most notably serotonin (5-HT) or substance P. The additional/excessive hormones lead to a wide range of symptoms called **"carcinoid syndrome"** which can significantly impact the quality of life for patients. Included among these symptoms are the following:
- flushing;
- diarrhea;
- asthma or wheezing;
- congestive heart failure (CHF);
- abdominal cramping;
- peripheral edema; and,
- heart palpitations.

Like many who learn they have this rare, incurable neuroendocrine cancer, after the initial shock wore off, I simply had to learn everything I could about this sinister cancer. This was not only to

MY JOURNEY WITH NEUROENDOCRINE CANCER
What You Don't Know Can Kill You!

better understand what I was up against, but also to learn what, if anything, I could do to fight it ... and outlive it.

What I discovered was a surprising mountain of useful, technical information on neuroendocrine cancer, synthetic somatostatin analogues, and so much more. Allow me to share the highlights of what I learned.

To begin, I first learned the very basics of how neuroendocrine cancer begins. When a cell grows abnormally, what it forms is called a tumor. When tumors spread within an organ or to other organs, it is said they have "metastasized," and they are then classified as "cancerous."

When a cancerous tumor occurs in the neuroendocrine system, it is called a neuroendocrine tumor or a NET. NETs grow slowly over many years and typically cause few, if any, symptoms until they become large, spread to other parts of the body ... or are located in a vital part of the body and cause noticeable physical difficulties. That is what happened to me. A NET located on my ampulla of vater eventually grew large enough to entirely close off that part of my digestive system!

With this general background, I set out to learn more about neuroendocrine cancer in terms of hormones and what they do in the body. I learned that hormones are produced in the endocrine system through cells and glands located throughout the body. Neuroendocrine cells (nerve cells) also make hormones. Hormones control vital functions in the body such as metabolism, appetite, and even our emotions. I was especially surprised to learn that nerve cells in our body actually communicate with each other through hormones!

My focus then turned to learning more about the specific hormone called serotonin. I learned it is a natural hormone mainly found in the brain, gut and blood platelets. In particular, it helps to control digestion, moods such as happiness and optimism, and it plays an important role in helping with movement along the digestive tract. After serotonin breaks down in the body, it normally is released in the urine as a chemical known as 5-HIAA.

When NETs become large or spread to other parts of the body, they produce and send out their own created serotonin hormone into the bloodstream. This results in far too much serotonin circulating in the body which, in turn, causes significant physical and emotional suffering in a number of ways referred to as, "Carcinoid Syndrome."

The next hormone I researched was somatostatin, a hormone that is naturally secreted at several locations in the digestive system. It is classified as an "inhibitory hormone" because it actually restrains the activity of certain pancreatic and gastrointestinal hormones. Somatostatin is found widely distributed throughout the central nervous system and it occurs in other tissues in the body.

Since somatostatin inhibits the actions of excessive amounts of serotonin in the body and reduces related debilitating effects, a synthetic somatostatin analogue is part of a treatment process for patients with neuroendocrine cancer.

Synthetic somatostatin analogue treatments are administered using either "Octreotide" (brand name "Sandostatin") produced by Novartis Pharmaceutical, or, "Somatuline" (brand name "Lanreotide") produced by Ipsen Pharmaceuticals. Sandostatin and Lanreotide medicines, owned and manufactured by French pharmaceuticals, have received FDA approval for use in the United States.

Both Sandostatin and Lanreotide pharmacologically mimic natural somatostatin, and in so doing, they reduce the harmful levels of excessive amounts of serotonin in the body caused by NETs. Since both analogues are poorly absorbed in the gut, they are administered subcutaneously, intramuscularly or intravenously. A three-inch needle is used intramuscularly to inject Sandostatin; a one-inch needle is used subcutaneously to inject Lanreotide.

Both synthetic somatostatin analogues are now widely used to medically treat patients who have neuroendocrine tumors. These analogues are seen as a method to reduce the unpleasant effects of carcinoid syndrome caused by neuroendocrine tumors. In some NET patients, these analogues have also been reported to stabilize or even reduce neuroendocrine tumors.

For the inhibition of somatostatin analogues to work effectively, there needs to be a route into the over-secreting tumors, normally via short or long acting injections or intravenously (IV). On tumor cells, there are currently five known Somatostatin Receptors which are expressed by most NETs. The SSA will attempt to bind with these receptors to inhibit certain hormones and peptides.

My next discovery involved learning more about something I had never heard of before … "biochemical markers." To begin, a biochemical marker is a measurable substance, or substances, which are produced and released from neuroendocrine tumor cells. These biochemical markers make it possible to gauge the level of tumor cell activity. Specifically, carcinoid tumor cells contain small clear vesicles that synthesize and release numerous potentially bioactive proteins and hormones including Chromogranin A, serotonin, Substance P, histamines, and Gastrin. These are some of the most common biochemical markers that are found evaluated in patients with neuroendocrine cancer.

The clinical significance of these neuroendocrine tumor biochemical markers is that they can assist in diagnosis and related evaluation. In particular, positive "Immunohistochemical staining" for Chromogranin (Cg), Synaptophysin, and Neuron Specific Enolase (NSE) provide evidence for a definitive diagnosis of a neuroendocrine tumor.

In addition, positive "Ki67 staining" gives a pathologist supporting evidence in grading the tumor. The pathologist begins by reviewing biopsy samples of the tumor under a microscope and in 10 high-powered fields. He attempts to count the cells undergoing "mitosis[14]." The number of cells actively dividing determines the relative "tumor grade."

Tumor grade is important in determining management of neuroendocrine cancer. A well-differentiated or low-grade tumor grows slower than a poorly differentiated or high-grade tumor.

Hormonal markers can also provide evidence of the site of origin for the primary tumor. This is especially helpful in cases where the cancer has metastasized and location of the primary tumor is unknown.

---

[14] **Mitosis** – This is the process by which a single cell divides into two cells. Synonyms include cell division, cell growth, or cell proliferation. Two cells are formed from a single parent cell. The new cells are identical to one another and to the original parent cell.

MY JOURNEY WITH NEUROENDOCRINE CANCER
What You Don't Know Can Kill You!

The sites are divided into three areas. Foregut is one area that includes bronchial, pancreatic, gastric and duodenal. Midgut is the area that includes the small bowel, ascending colon and part of transverse colon. Hindgut is the third area that includes the rest of transverse colon, descending and sigmoid and rectal colon.

Interestingly, there are differences in behavior of the neuroendocrine tumors depending on the site of origin based on differences in elevated hormonal expressions. They can express and cause different symptoms and metastasize to different areas. This is important when it comes to investigating the relative stage or the overall burden of the cancer.

BOB WALSH

Chapter 35

CARCINOID TUMORS

Carcinoid tumors are abnormal growths that begin in the neuroendocrine cells which are distributed widely throughout the body. Carcinoids are also referred to as "neuroendocrine tumors (NETs)."

Carcinoid tumors are the most commonly occurring gut endocrine tumors. The prevalence of carcinoids is about 50,000 cases in any one year in the United States. The incidence is estimated to be approximately 1.5 cases per 100,000 of the general population (i.e., approximately 2500 new cases per year in the United States). Nonetheless, they account for 13% to 34% of all tumors of the small bowel and 17% to 46% of all malignant tumors of the small bowel.

They derive from primitive stem cells generally found in the gut wall. Carcinoids may, however, occur in the bronchus, pancreas, rectum, ovary, lung and elsewhere.

The tumors grow slowly and often are clinically silent for many years before metastasizing. They frequently metastasize to the regional lymph nodes, liver, and, less commonly, to bone. The likelihood of metastases relates to tumor size. The incidence of metastases is less than 15% with a carcinoid tumor smaller than 1 cm but rises to 95% with tumors larger than 2 cm.

In individual cases, size alone may not be the only determinant of lymphatic or distant spread. Lymphatic or vascular invasion, or if the cancer has spread into the fat surrounding the primary tumor, this may be an indicator of a more aggressive tumor.

All this represents just the tip of the iceberg when it comes to neuroendocrine cancer.

Chapter 36

TYPES OF NEUROENDOCRINE TUMORS (NETS)

Neuroendocrine tumors (NETs) are considered the "zebras" of the cancer world because they behave so differently from other cancers.

Why zebras? Well, when you hear the hoof-beats of a zebra, they sound exactly like that of a horse but, of course, a zebra is completely different from a horse. Like hoof-beats, cancer symptoms often lead to misdiagnosing neuroendocrine cancer as some other type of cancer.

While NETs typically grow slowly, they can grow and spread in a stealth-like manner. They can be very small and develop anywhere in the body, such as the stomach, intestines, pancreas and lungs. Because they don't show up on typical PET scans, finding them at early stages and/or detecting metastasis is quite difficult.

While some features of neuroendocrine tumors are unique to the site of origin, other characteristics are shared, regardless of site. There are various types of neuroendocrine tumors that occur in different places in the body, and they grow differently.

Characteristics of neuroendocrine tumors include, in part:
- they are rare;
- usually small (< 1 cm);
- they grow slowly (months to years);
- usually found to metastasize to the liver and bone before becoming symptomatic - often when the tumor is larger than 2 cm;

- NETs may be silent for many years;
- often misdiagnosed since symptoms mimic commonplace conditions; and,
- diagnosis is rarely made clinically since neuroendocrine tumors require sophisticated laboratory and scanning techniques to identify.

Many NETs first appear in the lungs or the gastrointestinal tract, including the stomach, pancreas, appendix, intestines, colon and rectum. NETs may also appear in the thymus, thyroid gland, adrenal gland and pituitary gland. NETs may be classified by the site of their origin. Doctors may use terms such as "GI NET," "pancreatic NET" or "lung NET" to describe the tumor. Although NETs vary in size and how quickly they grow, almost all NETs are considered to be malignant or cancerous.

Although NETs comprise less than two percent of GI malignancies, these tumors are actually more prevalent than stomach and pancreatic cancers combined. Data from the National Cancer Institute (NCI) shows a five-fold increase in the incidence of neuroendocrine tumors from 1973 to 2004. The incidence of NETs has continued to rise and has, in fact, markedly increased over recent years.

Common neuroendocrine tumors (NETs) include:
- Carcinoid;
- Insulinoma;
- PPoma;
- Gastrinoma;
- VIPoma;
- Glucagonoma;

- Somatostatinoma
- Multiple Endocrine Neoplasia Types 1 and 2 (MEN-1 and MEN-2); and,
- Other rare tumors include Ghrelinoma.

The great majority of NETs are carcinoid tumors accounting for more than half of those presenting each year. The incidence of carcinoids has risen in recent years, especially those found in the stomach and ileum. Insulinomas, gastrinomas, and PPomas account for 17%, 15%, and 9% respectively, whereas the rest remain around the 1% mark.

Recent data suggests 60-80% of **pNETS** may not be functional or simply may not appear to be so … simply because the offending hormone or peptide has not yet been identified.

Gastric Neuroendocrine Tumors (gNets)

Although uncommon, the diagnosis of gNets is increasing due to the widespread use of upper digestive endoscopy. They are often visualized as small reddish polyps.

Type 1 Gastric Carcinoid Tumors

These tumors are associated with high gastrin levels, and multiple, small, relatively nonaggressive tumors. These tumors are accompanied by pernicious anemia and vitamin B12 deficiency in which there is loss of gastric acid secretion causing impairment of the normal restraint mechanism suppressing gastrin production.

Type 2 Gastric Carcinoid Tumors

These tumors are associated with elevated gastric acid, high gastrin levels, and the Zollinger-Ellison (ZE) syndrome. These tumors are larger and have a higher propensity to metastasize than type 1 carcinoids of the stomach.

Type 3 Gastric Carcinoid Tumors
These tumors are much larger than types 1 and 2 and have a high propensity to metastasize. These tumors are sporadic and may be associated with normal gastrin and gastric acid levels. This type of gastric carcinoid is most likely to cause tumor-related deaths.

Foregut Carcinoid Tumors
Sporadic primary foregut tumors include carcinoids of the bronchus, stomach, first portion of the duodenum, pancreas and ovaries. It is not unusual for foregut carcinoid tumors to metastasize to bone. These tumors are unusual for the following reasons:
- flushing tends to be of protracted duration;
- flushing is often purplish or violet instead of the usual pink or red; and,
- flushing frequently results in spider veins and enlargement of an organ or tissue from an increase in size of the cells of the skin of the face and upper neck.

Midgut Carcinoid Tumors
Midgut carcinoid tumors derive from the second portion of the duodenum, the jejunum, the ileum and the right colon. Midgut carcinoids have high serotonin content, rarely secrete 5-HTP, and often produce a number of other vasoactive compounds. The classic carcinoid syndrome includes flushing and diarrhea with or without wheezing. These tumors may produce adrenocorticotropic hormone (ACTH) on rare occasions and infrequently metastasize to bone.

Hindgut Carcinoid Tumors

Hindgut carcinoid tumors include those of the transverse colon, left colon, and rectum. This distinction assists in distinguishing a number of important biochemical and clinical differences among carcinoid tumors because the presentation, histochemistry, and secretory products are quite different.

Hindgut carcinoids rarely contain serotonin, rarely secrete 5-HTP or other peptides, and are usually silent in their presentation. However, they may metastasize to bone. A further point of interest is that a gender variation is present when a carcinoid tumor coexists with MEN-I; more than two-thirds of the time the tumor is in the thymus in males; whereas, in females, more than 75% of the time it is in the lung.

BOB WALSH

Chapter 37

SYMPTOMS OF NEUROENDOCRINE CANCER

Symptoms vary from patient to patient but can include vague abdominal pain, fatigue, wheezing, flushing and can even cause damage to heart valves. Unfortunately, many of these symptoms do not occur until the tumor has spread to the liver ... or the tumor begins to cause pain and/or other difficulties due to its location in the body.

Different types of NETs cause different symptoms, depending on the location of the tumor, and whether the NET is functional or nonfunctional. Functioning NETs are defined based upon the presence of clinical symptoms due to excess hormone secretion by the tumor. Nonfunctional NETs do not secrete hormones. They may produce symptoms caused by the tumor's growth.

Some of the more common symptoms of NETs include:
- Flushing (redness, warmth) in the face or neck without sweating;
- Diarrhea, including at nighttime;
- Shortness of breath, rapid heartbeat/palpitations;
- High blood pressure;
- Fatigue, weakness;
- Abdominal pain, cramping, feeling of fullness;
- Unexplained weight gain or loss;
- Wheezing, coughing;
- Swelling in the feet and ankles;
- Skin lesions, discolored patches of skin, thin skin;

- High blood glucose levels (frequent urination, increased thirst, increased hunger); and,
- Low blood glucose levels (shakiness, dizziness, sweating and fainting.)

Frequency of clinical manifestations of symptoms reflecting neuroendocrine tumors

- Flushing — 84%
- Diarrhea — 79%
- Hypertension* — 50%
- Bronchoconstriction — 17%
- Heart disease* — <10%
- Myopathy — 7%
- Pigmentation — 5%
- Arthropathy — 5%
- Hyper-hypoglycemia — <1%
- Ulcer disease — <1%
- Dermopathy — <1%

* **Note**: The incidence of right-sided valvular heart disease has markedly decreased over recent decades since the widespread use of somatostatin analogs. However, over the same time period, the incidence of hypertension has increased.

NETs often do not cause symptoms early in the disease process. When symptoms are present, they may be similar to those caused by more common conditions. As a result, NETs are sometimes misdiagnosed as irritable bowel syndrome (IBS). However, with IBS, abdominal discomfort is usually relieved by going to the bathroom.

Since most NET patients are diagnosed at a late stage, it's important for the patient to let the doctor know if new or persisting symptoms or changes are noticed in his body.

Symptom of Neuroendocrine Cancer: Flushing

Flushing is a cardinal symptom of carcinoid tumors but also occurs in a variety of other conditions. A good rule of thumb is if the flushing is **"wet"** (that is, accompanied by sweating), it is due to a cause other than to carcinoid.

Distinguishing Signs and Symptoms

There are two varieties of flushing related to carcinoid syndrome.

1. Midgut carcinoid: The flushing usually is faint pink to red in color and involves the face and upper trunk as far as the nipple line. The flush is initially provoked by alcohol and food containing tyramine (e.g., blue cheese, chocolate, aged or cured sausage, red wine). With time, the flush may occur spontaneously and without provocation. It usually lasts only a few minutes and may occur many times per day. It generally does not leave permanent discoloration.

2. Foregut tumors: The flushing often is more intense, of longer duration, and purplish in hue. It is frequently followed by spider veins and involves the upper trunk and may also affect the limbs.

Hormones and Peptides

Tests are conducted to measure the levels of hormones and peptides ascribed to flushing in carcinoid syndrome. Among these tests are:
- 5-HIAA (plasma or urine);
- Calcitonin;

- Gastrin;
- Gastrin-releasing peptide (GRP);
- Prostaglandins;
- Serotonin (5-HT);
- Somatostatin;
- Substance P;
- Vasoactive neuropeptides (serotonin, dopamine, histamine); and,
- Vasoactive Intestinal Polypeptide (VIP).

Symptom of Neuroendocrine Cancer: Diarrhea

Watery diarrhea syndrome (WDHHA), caused by a pancreatic islet cell tumor, was first identified in 1958. As implied by its name, the primary characteristic is watery diarrhea.

A critical distinguishing difference from the Zollinger-Ellison (ZE) syndrome is the absence of hyperacidity and the marked presence of hypokalemia[15]. Diarrhea in the Zollinger-Ellison (ZE) syndrome improves with inhibition of acid secretion, whereas in WDHHA it does not.

The WDHHA usually begins with intermittent diarrhea, but as the tumor grows, the episodic diarrhea becomes continuous and persists despite fasting (i.e., it is secretory, not malabsorptive).

Hypercalcemia occurs in WDHHA because of direct effects of VIP on bone. It is important to differentiate this cause of hypercalcemia from the hypercalcemia caused by excess PTH release from

---

[15] **Hypokalemia** – This is when blood's potassium levels are too low. Potassium is an important electrolyte for nerve and muscle cell functioning, especially for muscle cells in the heart. The kidneys control the body's potassium levels, allowing for excess potassium to leave the body through urine or sweat.

parathyroid glands seen in the sporadic (usually caused by adenomas) or familial (usually the result of hyperplastic glands) forms of hyperthyroidism.

Distinguishing Signs and Symptoms
- Profuse diarrhea with the appearance of weak tea;
- Presence of marked hypokalemia and hyperchloremic acidosis;
- Initial intermittent diarrhea, becoming continuous as tumor grows;
- Secretory nature of diarrhea (i.e., does not disappear even after fasting for 48 hours);
- Absence of gastric hyperacidity (a major feature distinguishing WDHHA from the Zollinger-Ellison (ZE) syndrome);
- Atrophic gastritis or pernicious anemia or gastric carcinoid type 1;
- Hypochlorhydria resulting from the gastric inhibitory effect of VIP;
- Secretion of HCO3 and causes life-threatening loss of electrolytes into the stool;
- Increased intestinal motility as well as secretion adding to the diarrhea;
- Hypercalcemia not due to PTH or PTHrp;
- Hyperglycemia or abnormal glucose tolerance;
- Dilation of the gallbladder;
- Flushing;
- Weight loss; and,
- Colic.

Patients with watery diarrhea are often severely dehydrated, and their fluid balance and electrolytes should be corrected before specific diagnostic tests are initiated, except for evaluation of stool electrolytes and concentration of a solution expressed as the total number of solute particles per liter.

Diagnostic Tests
- Exclude atrophic gastritis, pernicious anemia, and gastric carcinoid;
- Exclude use of proton pump inhibitors;
- Exclude the Zollinger-Ellison (ZE) syndrome;
- Determine the probability of a pancreatic-based source of watery diarrhea (VIP, Pancreatic Polypeptide(PP), MCT, CT, and OctreoScan®); and,
- Eliminate other syndromes masquerading as WDHHA and producing similar symptoms.

Hormones and Peptides
Vasoactive intestinal polypeptide is the primary peptide produced by the majority of pancreatic tumors (VIPomas) causing WDHHA. Because VIP is also produced by neural cells, elevated levels of other GI and pancreatic hormones and peptides may be markers for establishing the presence of a pancreatic tumor associated with diarrhea.

Symptom of Neuroendocrine Cancer: Endocrine Hypertension
A possible cause of hypertension - elevated blood pressure - may be related to carcinoid syndrome. Proper testing by a patient's medical team can help to determine if the hypertension may be related to NET cancer.

Symptom of Neuroendocrine Cancer: Wheezing

A possible cause of wheezing may be related to carcinoid syndrome. Proper testing by a patient's medical team can help to determine if the hypertension may be related to NET cancer.

BOB WALSH

Chapter 38

THE CARCINOID SYNDROME

The carcinoid syndrome occurs in less than 10% of patients who have carcinoid tumors. It is especially common in tumors of the ileum and jejunum (i.e., midgut tumors) but also occurs with bronchial, ovarian and other carcinoids. Tumors in the rectum (i.e., hindgut tumors) rarely produce the carcinoid syndrome, even those that have widely metastasized.

Tumors may be symptomatic only episodically, and their existence may go unrecognized for many years. The average time from onset of symptoms attributable to the tumor and diagnosis is just over 9 years, and diagnosis usually is made only after the carcinoid syndrome occurs.

The distribution of carcinoids is **Gaussian**[16] in nature. The peak incidence occurs in the sixth and seventh decades of life, but carcinoid tumors have also been reported in patients as young as 10 years of age and in those in their ninth decade. There is an overall increase in incidence of carcinoid tumors over recent years.

During the early stages, vague abdominal pain goes undiagnosed and invariably is ascribed to irritable bowel or spastic colon. At least one-third of patients with small bowel carcinoid tumors experience several years of intermittent abdominal pain before diagnosis. This pain can be due to obstruction (partial or

---

[16] **Gaussian** - In probability theory, the normal (or Gaussian or Gauss or Laplace-Gauss) distribution is a very common continuous probability distribution. Normal distributions are important in statistics and are often used in the natural and social sciences to represent real-valued random variables whose distributions are not known.

intermittent) or to the development of intestinal angina, which in turn, may be due to bowel **ischemia**[17], especially after eating.

Carcinoid tumors can present in a variety of ways. For example, duodenal tumors are known to produce gastrin and may present with the gastrinoma syndrome[18]. One of the more clinically useful classifications of carcinoid tumors is according to the classification of the primitive gut from which the tumor cells arise. These tumors derive from the stomach, foregut, midgut, and hindgut.

---

[17] **Ischemia** – This is a restriction in blood supply to tissues, causing a shortage of oxygen that is needed for cellular metabolism (to keep tissue alive). Ischemia is generally caused by problems with blood vessels, with resultant damage to - or dysfunction - of tissue.
[18] **Gastrinoma Syndrome** – A gastrinoma is a type of pancreatic neuroendocrine tumor, which is a rare endocrine tumor that occurs sporadically as well as part of inherited familial endocrine syndromes such as Multiple Endocrine Neoplasia Type-1 (MEN-1).

MY JOURNEY WITH NEUROENDOCRINE CANCER
What You Don't Know Can Kill You!

Chapter 39

CARCINOID CRISIS

A carcinoid crisis involves profound flushing, bronchospasm, tachycardia, and widely and rapidly fluctuating blood pressure. It can occur when large amounts of hormone are acutely secreted as occasionally triggered by factors such as diet, alcohol, surgery chemotherapy, embolization therapy or radiofrequency ablation.

Chronic exposure to high levels of serotonin causes thickening of the heart valves, particularly the tricuspid and the pulmonic valves, and over a long period can lead to congestive heart failure. However, valve replacement is rarely needed. The excessive outflow of serotonin can cause a depletion of tryptophan leading to niacin deficiency, and thus pellagra, which is associated with dermatitis, dementia and diarrhea.

Many other hormones can be secreted by some of these tumors, most commonly growth hormone that can cause acromegaly, or cortisol, that can cause Cushing's syndrome[19]. Occasionally, hemorrhage or the effects of tumor bulk are the presenting symptoms. Bowel obstruction can occur, sometimes due to the fibrosing effects of neuroendocrine cancer.

---

[19] **Cushing Syndrome** – This is a primary adrenal gland disease. In some people, the cause of Cushing Syndrome is excess cortisol secretion that doesn't depend on stimulation from ACTH and is associated with disorders of the adrenal glands. The most common of these disorders is a noncancerous tumor of the adrenal cortex, called an adrenal adenoma.

BOB WALSH

Chapter 40

TREATING NEUROENDOCRINE CANCER

A treatment plan for neuroendocrine cancer is highly individualized. The relevant considerations, in part, include the following:
- Location of the tumor;
- whether it has metastasized; and,
- if the patient suffers from carcinoid syndrome.

In addition, identifying the particular stage of disease is a vital step in structuring the appropriate treatment for neuroendocrine cancer. This considers if the NETs are:
- contained in a particular area of the body (localized); or,
- have spread to nearby tissues and/or lymph nodes (regional); and/or,
- have spread throughout the body (metastatic).

In over 50% of the cases, it is estimated that NETs have already spread to other parts of the body by the time they are diagnosed. NETs metastasize most often to the liver, peritoneal cavity or to the bone.

Neuroendocrine tumors are staged according to the "TNM Staging System" which considers the following:
- the tumor (T);
- the node (N); and,
- the metastasis (M).

The World Health Organization (WHO) classifies neuroendocrine tumors according to the particular malignant potential of the tumor. For example:
- well-differentiated neuroendocrine tumors are grade 1 and 2; and,
- poorly-differentiated neuroendocrine tumors are considered grade 3.

There are many types of neuroendocrine tumors, and each requires a different approach to diagnosis and treatment. Diagnosis of NETs generally depends upon the following conditions:
- the type of tumor;
- its location;
- whether the tumor produces excess hormones;
- how aggressive it is; and,
- if the tumor has spread to other areas of the body.

Oncologists use diagnostic tools to evaluate the disease and structure the individualized treatment plan accordingly. Among the tests which can be used in diagnosis, are the following:
- lab tests, cytopathology;
- biopsy, endoscopic ultrasound;
- ERCP;
- CT scan, CT angiography;
- MRI;
- laparoscopy;
- nuclear medicine imaging; and,
- genetic testing and counseling.

Positron Emission Tomography (PET) scans can detect cancer by infusing the patient with a glucose preparation and then identifying the body areas where the glucose is consumed or metabolized abnormally fast.

Since most NETs do not consume glucose rapidly, an agent called "Gallium-68 Dota-tate" can be used as a PET scan tracer (rather than using glucose) to identify carcinoid tumors including very small lesions. Results using Gallium-68 Dota-tate have been reported as significantly better than other imaging techniques. Gallium-68 Dota-tate has FDA approval.

While NETs do not consume glucose as other cancers do, their cells have many receptors for a hormone, "somatostatin," which regulates the endocrine system. Gallium-68 Dota-tate is a radioactive look-alike of the hormone that can bind to the somatostatin receptors, and when it does, it highlights NET tumors so they can be seen on PET scan imaging.

This imaging technique significantly improves the detection of NETs in three important ways:
- <u>Faster process</u>. The process is completed in a few hours. This test is much quicker than the three-day "OctreoScan" which uses a different radioactive drug and a gamma camera to measure the radio material over time.
- <u>Better images</u>. Because of the high sensitivity and combining of PET with CT, physicians are able to get a very clear, high-resolution image that can identify very small lesions which otherwise would be missed.
- <u>Guides treatment</u>. The improved imaging helps oncologists choose an optimal therapy - such as surgery versus systemic therapy.

Once a diagnosis of neuroendocrine cancer is made, oncologists and their teams can work with the cancer patient to develop a comprehensive treatment plan based on the patient's unique diagnosis and needs.

Since most NET patients are diagnosed at a late stage, an integrative approach is essential to each patient's treatment and care. The patient's team of collaborative cancer care professionals has two primary goals when designing the treatment plan:
- attack the cancer itself; and,
- combat the cancer-related side effects.

The treatment plan for neuroendocrine cancer varies depending upon each patient's specific factors (such as type and stage of the cancer.) Listed below are some of the more common treatment options which can be used when treating patients with NET tumors.

- **Surgery:** Surgical removal of the primary tumor is often the first option for patients with localized NETs. The goal of surgery can be to fully remove the NET tumor, or to reduce the tumor's "burden." Surgery may also be an option for those with advanced disease to help relieve some of the symptoms of neuroendocrine cancer. Surgical procedures for NETs can include debulking or cytoreductive surgery, minimally invasive laparoscopic resections, and liver transplantation.

- **Medical oncology:** Depending upon the specific type of neuroendocrine cancer and the treatment goals, chemotherapy, hormone therapy and/or targeted therapy may be used to manage certain types of NETs - including advanced NETs. Some targeted therapies for pancreatic NETs may include use of chemotherapy drugs administered directly into the NET tumor. This may be an option in cases where the disease has metastasized to the liver.

- **Radiation oncology:** Radiation therapy is generally used when a neuroendocrine tumor has spread - or is in a location that makes surgical options difficult. Such a therapy is a non-invasive option for neuroendocrine cancer patients. It enables radiation oncologists to deliver high, targeted doses of radiation to the NET tumors. For metastatic disease to the liver, this therapy delivers radiation directly to NET tumors in the liver.

- **Interventional radiology:** Radiofrequency ablation (a form of surgical removal) may be used for NETs that have spread to the liver. This technique uses high-energy radio waves to heat and destroy the cancerous cells. This is a minimally invasive option for patients with inoperable tumors – or those that are difficult to reach. Instead of using extreme heat or cold which may damage normal adjacent tissue, interventional radiology uses electrical currents to destroy NETs. For NETs which have spread to the liver, embolization techniques may help to reduce, or cut off, the supply of blood to the tumor.

- **Gastrointestinal procedures:** This plan can include a full range of treatment options for gastrointestinal NETs including technologies that involve minimally invasive ways. Such techniques and ablative treatments may help to remove obstructions in the gastrointestinal tract, and relieve pain and/or breathing problems.

- **Pain management:** Pain management and palliative care are essential parts of a treatment and care plan for patients with NETs. While the treatment plan is carried out, it is helpful if the pain management team is available to assist the patient in terms of anticipating - and proactively managing - related pain.

  The pain management team can also help the patient manage the possible side effects of pain medications - nausea, drowsiness, constipation, et al. The challenge is to find a balance between controlling related pain and preserving the quality of life for the cancer patient.

- **Nutrition therapy:** Nutrition is a very important part of the treatment plan dealing with neuroendocrine cancer. The tumors, particularly gastrointestinal NETs, can affect the body's ability to digest and absorb vital nutrients from food. This can put patients at risk for malnutrition.

  Symptoms may include nausea, taste changes, weight loss, fatigue, decreased appetite, fullness, pain, gas, diarrhea and constipation. The nutrition team can offer strategies designed to help the patient stay strong and properly nourished.

Nutrition therapy goals should be personalized for each cancer patient and be aimed at the achieving the following goals:
1. preventing or reversing poor nutrition;
2. managing nutrition-related symptoms; and,
3. maintaining or improving weight and strength.

Naturopathic medicine[20] Throughout treatment, neuroendocrine cancer patients may experience symptoms or discomfort after eating which may interfere with patients' ability to digest nutrients and fat-soluble vitamins. Naturopathic clinicians can work with the neuroendocrine cancer patients' oncologists to recommend a variety of supplements and botanicals designed to offer upper gastrointestinal health.

Such naturopathic therapies may also help neuroendocrine cancer patients in other important ways:
1. manage endocrine and blood sugar abnormalities;
2. digest food more easily;
3. better absorb nutrients;
4. help prevent and treat nausea; and,
5. reduce acid reflux, heartburn, bloating, gas and diarrhea.

---

[20] **Naturopathic medicine** is a distinct primary health care profession, emphasizing prevention, treatment, and optimal health through the use of therapeutic methods and substances that encourage individuals' inherent self-healing process. The practice of naturopathic medicine includes modern and traditional, scientific, and empirical methods.

BOB WALSH

Chapter 41

PEPTIDE RECEPTOR RADIONUCLIDE THERAPY (PRRT)

Peptide Receptor Radionuclide Therapy (PRRT) is a form of molecular-targeted therapy that is performed by using a small peptide (a somatostatin analog similar to octreotide) coupled with a radionuclide emitting beta radiation.

PRRT is a nuclear medicine therapy (the first patients were treated in 1996) for the systemic treatment of metastasized neuroendocrine tumors. These types of tumors include gastroenteropancreatic tumors (so **call**ed GEP-NETs), e.g. arising from the small bowel (often called carcinoid tumors), the pancreas, duodenum or stomach, but also from the large bowel or the lung and many other tissues (so called "diffuse neuroendocrine system").

A handful of medical centers in Europe have been doing PRRT since the mid-1990s including Basel, Milano, Rotterdam and Bad Berka[21]. A clinical trial on PRRT began in the United States with Lutetium-177 Dota-tate in 2013, and on January 26, 2018, was approved by the US Food and Drug Administration.

A helpful way to understand how PRRT works is to consider a type of "Trojan Horse" packed with cancer-killing radiation inside. Also, think of PRRT like a magnet with the ability to attract iron shavings:
1. Think of a neuroendocrine tumor with somatostatin positive receptors as the magnet;

---

[21] **Bad Berka** – This is a German city situated in the south of the Weimar region in the state of Thuringia. With almost 8,000 inhabitants, Bad Berka is the second biggest city in the Weimarer Land district.

2. Think of iron shavings as a somatostatin analog chemical (Octreotide) to which is bound or attached to some radioactive material (the radionuclide Y90 or LU177);
3. The receptors in the tumors attract the octreotide and this chemical with the radioactive material is absorbed into the tumor by the receptors; and,
4. **The radiation then starts to kill the tumor cells!**

It is important to note that Peptide Receptor Radionuclide Therapy (PRRT) does **NOT** work on all neuroendocrine tumors. For this treatment to work, the patient MUST have somatostatin receptors in his/her tumors. When a somatostatin analog (like a form of Octreotide) is combined with a radionuclide such as Lutetium-177 (LU177) or Yttrium-90 (Y90), it has a strong affinity for the somatostatin receptor subtype-2 which can exist in a NET tumor.

This means that the radioactive material put in the body for the treatment will be absorbed directly by the NET tumor that has the receptor. When the radioactive material is thus absorbed into the NET tumor, the tumor dies.

PRRT is considered a systemic form of treatment that can affect neuroendocrine tumors with receptors wherever they may be located in the body. This form of treatment is used primarily for cancer patients with tumors that cannot be removed through surgery in multiple sites. Other patients who have neuroendocrine tumors only in the liver are treated with this therapy in order to reduce the size and number of the NETs present in the liver or in other areas of the body in preparation for subsequent surgery.

In addition to needing somatostatin receptors in a patient's tumors, other factors must be weighed before a decision is made to pursue this form of treatment. Such factors include "tumor load" in terms of size, number of tumors and location of tumors. Other important considerations include the age of the patient and his/her physical condition. It has been reported that patients taking long-acting somatostatin analogues (for example, Sandostatin) should delay this particular test for three to four weeks after their last dose.

As with most treatment options available to neuroendocrine cancer patients, there are risks associated with using PRRT to treat metastasized NETs. The greatest risks are associated with radiation toxicity affecting three key areas:
- the blood system (producing red blood cells, white blood cells and blood platelets);
- functioning of the kidneys; and,
- functioning of the liver.

At one time, kidney impairment or renal insufficiency was a regarded as a significant risk, however, as methods of protecting the kidneys during PRRT became better refined, this risk has been diminished. Medical centers administering PRRT are now reported to initiate specific measures to protect the kidneys using forms of amino acids infused before and after treatment. As of this writing in 2018, specific protective measures have not been developed for the liver or blood system. Better control over radiation dosage helps to reduce toxicity from the radiation.

Each patient is different in terms of how they react to PRRT but there are some side-effects commonly observed among patients. The duration of these side effects varies greatly from a few hours to several days.

Common side-effects of PRRT have been reported to include:
- Nausea;
- Vomiting; and,
- Abdominal discomfort or pain.

Less common side-effects of PRRT have been reported are:
- Subacute hematological toxicity; and,
- Temporary hair loss.

In some cases, it has also been reported that PRRT patients have experienced delayed toxicity to the kidneys, and renal insufficiency. Serious hematologic toxicity is rare.

According to the "Neuroendocrine Tumor Research Foundation" (netrf.org) in August 2018, common side effects of Lu-177 include:
- Low levels of white blood cells;
- High levels of enzymes in certain organs;
- Vomiting;
- Nausea;
- High levels of blood sugar;
- Low levels of potassium in the blood'
- Low levels of blood cells;
- Development of certain blood or bone marrow cancers;
- Kidney damage;
- Liver damage; and,
- Abnormal hormones levels."

In terms of results, most cancer patients typically want to understand the statistics associated with survival for their particular form of cancer. The survival rate and other measures in terms of months or years is almost always part of any report on the efficacy

MY JOURNEY WITH NEUROENDOCRINE CANCER
What You Don't Know Can Kill You!

of a particular treatment. For patients being treated for neuroendocrine cancer, there are several measures of treatment efficacy that are important when considering a treatment plan.

When evaluating which treatment plan is right for the neuroendocrine cancer patient, it is helpful to compare the "Time to Progression/Progression Free Survival" and "Duration of Therapy Response" for PRRT to other modalities under consideration.

Also of interest is the measurement referred to as, "Overall Survival" (OS). From a NET cancer patient's perspective, this may be the most important statistic to know and understand. It is the amount of time between when treatment begins and when the tumor/tumors start to grow - or new ones are found.

The best a cancer patient can do is to treat the cancer as if it is a chronic illness. This means using a treatment plan to stabilize or even reduce the tumors in the body, and then repeat the treatment - or go to a different plan to attack the tumors once they start growing and/or reappearing. This measurement, often expressed in terms of months, has been called the "Median Time to Progression."

In terms of comparing PRRT to chemotherapy, according to the article published by Dr. Kwekkeboom and colleagues in January of 2010 on PRRT, the median time for progression for most studies on chemotherapy shows less than 18 months. By comparison, the median time to progression for PRRT with Y-90 was 30 months, and with Lu-177, 40 months.

In terms of the Duration of Therapy response, once PRRT with either Y-90 or Lu-177 is used, the cell death process continues to work for a long which can be measured in terms of months. This is called the "Duration of Therapy Response." One treatment of PRRT is reported to be effective for more than two years during which time PRRT continues to cause neuroendocrine tumors to regress and die.

In studies by Dr. Kwekkeboom and his colleagues, the Duration of Therapy response for Y-90 octreotide and for Lu-177 octreotide was reported to be more than 30 months.

"Overall Survival" is another time-based measure that starts at the time of diagnosis, and covers the time for treatment until death. In most cases, this measurement pertains to a type of cancer. It is also being used to assess a patient's longevity once a particular type of treatment has been used.

In research published by Dr. Kwekkeboom and colleagues at Rotterdam, it was reported that overall survival for patients treated with Lu-177 Octreotide ranged from a low of 40 months to a high of 72 months from the time of diagnosis. Research by Dr. Richard Baum and colleagues at Bad Berka indicated the median overall survival was 59 months for 415 PRRT patients who were treated with a combination of Y-90 **and** Lu-177.

Chapter 42

INFORMATION RESOURCES ON THE INTERNET

ACOR
www.acor.org
Association of Cancer Online Resources. This is a forum for threaded discussions related to carcinoid cancer.

American Cancer Society
www.cancer.org

American Institute for Cancer Research
www.aicr.org
The New American Plate and Nutrition Information Center

Asia Pacific CNETs
www.cnets.org
Carcinoid Foundation from Singapore. This includes videos and patient information by physicians.

Australia
www.carcinoid.com/au
Provides "carcinoid cancer resources for Australians.

Australia Unicorn Foundation
www.unicornfoundation.org/au
This foundation is an Australian not-for-profit medical charity focused on neuroendocrine tumors (NET).

Board and Web Site
www.netpatientfoundation.com
This is a European based discussion board to discuss treatments available in Europe.

Breakaway from Cancer
www.breakawayfromcancer.com
This includes resources on preventing, fighting and surviving cancer.

Cancer Adventures
www.canceradventures.org
This website addresses ways to help cancer survivors meet their needs in terms of inspiration, nutrition and other resources for establishing their survivorship program.

CancerCare, Inc.
www.cancercare.org
800-813-HOPE
CancerCare is a national non-profit organization providing free professional support services to anyone affected by cancer. Included is information on care giving.

American Society of Clinical Oncology (ASCO)
www.cancer.net
ASCO provides oncologist-approved information about cancer. The website is available in English and Spanish.

Carcinoid Cancer Awareness Network
www.carcinoidawareness.org
Provides support and information for NET patients and their caregivers, and conducts national conferences that are available to be viewed online through webinars.

Carcinoid Cancer Foundation
www.carcinoid.org
Mission statement: "The Carcinoid Cancer Foundation is the oldest nonprofit carcinoid/and related neuroendocrine tumor organization in the United States, founded in 1968. The mission of this foundation is to increase awareness and educate the general public and healthcare professionals regarding carcinoid and related neuroendocrine tumors (NETs), to support NET cancer patients and their families, and to serve as patient advocates."

In summary, the Foundation which was founded in 1968:
- Provides information and educational materials for medical professionals, patients, and caregivers
- Provides e-mail and toll-free telephone support
- Continually works to improve access to accurate and up-to-date information
- Serves as advocates for the carcinoid/NET community
- Encourages research
- Participates as one of the founding members in the International Neuroendocrine Cancer Alliance (INCA)
- Created a carcinoid and neuroendocrine tumor database of approximately 2000 entries

Includes information about NET/carcinoid focused doctors around the globe, nutritional considerations, listing of community support groups, treatment, clinical trials and a wide variety of resources.

Caring for Carcinoid Foundation
www.caringforcarcinoid.org
Dedicated to funding and discovering cures for NETs, resources, physician database, research, announcements of latest advancements and research.

Clinical Trials
www.clinicaltrials.gov
US Government website detailing clinical trials.

CNETS Canada
Carcinoid Neuroendocrine Tumor Society
www.cnetscanada.org

ENETS
www.neuroendorcrine.net
Its mission statement: "Neuroendocrine tumors (NETs) present numerous complex clinical problems. Due to their relatively rare occurrence, research and patient care guidelines since the 1990s have been lacking. As a result, the European Neuroendocrine Tumor Society was founded in 2004 and the society members, currently numbering nearly 1,200, bring a variety of expertise from such fields as oncology, pathology, radiology, nuclear medicine, endocrinology, surgery and gastroenterology to ENETS.

ENETS goals include:
- Improve the diagnosis and therapy of patients with neuroendocrine tumors in an international, interdisciplinary and scientific context;
- Coordinate research at European hospitals and health research institutes, with emphasis on basic and clinical

research for the diagnosis and treatment of NETs;
- Further develop standards for the accreditations of ENETS Centers of Excellence;
- Offer education and training for physicians and scientists at annual scientific and educational meetings;
- Focus on writing and updating NET guidelines for all aspects of NET care including treatment and standards of care and subsequently publicizing in medical and scientific journals;
- Foster the exchange of forums for young investigators;
- Support collaborative scientific projects of excellence;
- Communicate with and inform patient advocates and patient self-help groups;
- Cooperate with the pharmaceutical industry for the development of new diagnostic, therapeutic and information technologies; and,
- Further endorse the ENETS Registry and Centers of Excellence throughout Europe.

InterScience Institute
www.interscienceinstitute.com

Live Strong
www.livestrong.org
Lance Armstrong's Foundation helps people with cancer and their loved ones through advocacy, education, public health and research.

Lucy's Blog
www.lucynoidblog.blogspot.com
Lucy, a carcinoid patient posts information and insight relevant for NET cancer patients.

Medline
www.nlm.nih.gov/medlineplus/
Comprehensive medical dictionary run by the National Institutes of Health (NIH)

Memorial Sloan-Kettering Cancer Center
www.mskcc.org/cancer-care
Help for caregivers, families and friends

NANETs North American Neuroendocrine Tumor Society
www.nanets.net
US NET/carcinoid medical society whose purpose is to improve neuroendocrine tumor (NET) disease management through increased research and educational opportunities. Coordinated by US carcinoid physicians.

National Cancer Association
www.nccn.org
Devoted to patients, caregivers and family, the only patient-oriented cancer website based on the NCCN Guidelines which set the standard of care of clinicians around the world.

National Cancer Institute Caregiver Information
http://cancer.gov

National Coalition for Cancer Survivorship
www.canceradvocacy.org
Information and resources on cancer support, advocacy and quality of life issues.

MY JOURNEY WITH NEUROENDOCRINE CANCER
What You Don't Know Can Kill You!

NET ALLIANCE
www.thenetalliance.com
Information, support and insights for people affected by neuroendocrine tumors. A Novartis Pharmaceutical sponsored site.

NET Patient Foundation
www.netpatientfoundation.com
Downloadable booklets, information, resources, physician database for USA and UK/Europe, links. Sponsored by pharmaceutical companies.

Patient Advocate Foundation
www.patientadvocate.org
Education, legal counseling and referrals to survivors concerning managed care, insurance, financial issues, job description, and debt crisis issues.

Society for Caring
www.strengthforcaring.com
This site is owned by Johnson & Johnson.

Sunny Susan Anderson
www.carcinoidinfo.info
The first personal website by a carcinoid patient, details her journey through carcinoid with educational resources available.

The Cancer Info Website
www.cancerlinksusa.com
Includes links to financial help organizations, recommendations for first steps after diagnosis, medical oncology terms dictionary.

The Insurance Warrior
www.theinsurancewarrior.com
Laurie Todd is a health insurance strategist. She writes insurance appeals. Her site offers tips on researching, writing, and delivery a winning appeal, offers appeal-writing services. She has written two books on the subject.

The Wellness Community
www.thewellnesscommunity.org

U.S. Department of Agriculture
www.fnic.nal.usda.gov
National Agriculture Library, Food

U.S. Food and Drug Administration
www.fda.gov

Yahoo Groups
www.groups.yahoo.com/group/CARCINOID-ACOR
A treaded discussion group for carcinoid education. Registration required. Monitored by Dr. Woltering at LSU-Kenner.

The National Organization for Rare Disorders
www.rarediseases.org
This is an alliance of health organizations which maintain a database with information about a multitude of rare diseases and related health advocacy and information groups.

The National Institutes of Health's (NIH) Office of Rare Disease Research
www.rarediseases.info.nih.gov
NIH offers an online gateway to a host of information links related to rare diseases, including rare cancers.

Carcinoid Coffee Cafe
https://www.facebook.com/Carcinoid/
This is a Carcinoid Cancer support group available on Facebook.

BOB WALSH

MY JOURNEY WITH NEUROENDOCRINE CANCER
What You Don't Know Can Kill You!

GLOSSARY

NEUROENDOCRINE CANCER TERMS

AUTHOR NOTE:
The items listed in this glossary were gathered from a number of different sources. In all cases, readers are encouraged to:
- Refer to your health care providers to confirm the meaning and significance of each item in this glossary – as well as those found in other areas of this book; and,
- Seek the advice and guidance of your physicians when dealing with any health issue.

5-HIAA – This is a breakdown-product of serotonin that is excreted in urine. Both serotonin and 5-HIAA are often found elevated in carcinoid patients.

Adrenal Glands – These endocrine glands are found located above each kidney. They secrete various hormones (like epinephrine and norepinephrine.)

Bile – This refers to a fluid produced by the liver. It is stored in the gallbladder. The function of bile is to aid in the digestion process.

Carcinoid – This is a term that describes slow growing tumors. Carcinoids can be categorized as being benign or malignant - or a combination of both. This has been referred to as "cancer in slow motion."

Carcinoid Crisis – This refers to when there is sudden flushing, and a change in blood pressure (usually a sudden drop in blood pressure, but it can also spike). This is can be brought on by stress or while the neuroendocrine cancer patient is under anesthesia.

Carcinoid Syndrome – This is a term used to describe a variety of symptoms caused by the release of serotonin and other substances from carcinoid tumors of the gastrointestinal tract. Symptoms can include diarrhea, bronchial spasms, flushing of the face, flat angiomas (small collections of dilated blood vessels) of the skin, rapid pulse and sudden drops in blood pressure.

Carcinoma – This refers to a type of cancer that starts in cells making up the skin or tissue lining organs. Like other types of cancer, carcinomas are abnormal cells that divide without control, and are able to spread to other parts of the body – but do not always. Some examples of carcinoma include the breast, colon, liver, pancreas, prostate or stomach.

Catheter – A catheter is a small, hollow tube that allows fluid passage. It is can aid diagnosis or specific medical procedures.

Chromogranin A – This is a "blood tumor marker" used to screen for various neuroendocrine tumors.

Cryoblation – This refers to a treatment designed to eliminate - or reduce - tumors by freezing the tumors using special instruments.

Depot Injection – A depot injection is a type of injection used that allows a substance injected at the original site to be absorbed by the body over an extended period of time.

MY JOURNEY WITH NEUROENDOCRINE CANCER
What You Don't Know Can Kill You!

Diuretic – A diuretic is a drug used to increase the flow of urine.

Dopamine – A dopamine is a neurotransmitter. It is formed in the brain and is necessary for the normal functioning of the body's central nervous system.

Endocrine System – The endocrine system consists of a series of glands that secrete numerous hormones.

Endoscope – An endoscope is an instrument that allows visual examination of internal organs (such as the stomach and colon).

Endoscopy – An endoscopy is a nonsurgical procedure that is used to examine a person's digestive tract. Using an endoscope (a flexible tube with a light and camera attached), the doctor can view pictures of the patient's digestive tract on a color monitor.

Gastrin – This is the name given for hormones that are secreted in the stomach and regulate gastric acid secretion.

Glucagon – This is the name of a hormone that is produced by the pancreas. Glucagon increases blood sugar levels.

Hepatic Artery – This is the artery that provides about 25% of the total blood supply to the liver - and 100% of the blood supply that nourishes tumors in the liver.

Hepatic Artery Chemo-Embolization – This is the term that describes the process whereby a catheter injects chemotherapy drugs directly into the hepatic artery thereby eliminating the blood supply to the liver and locking in the chemotherapy drugs.

Histamine – A histamine is a compound that is released by cells throughout the body as part of the body's inflammatory response to an infection, allergy or injury. When damaged or exposed to allergens[22], cells in the skin, nose, lungs and throat release histamine resulting in itchiness, pain, redness, runny nose and/or wheezing.

Hormones – A hormone is a substance produced by certain organs or cells and carried throughout the body via the bloodstream.

Hypokalemia – This is a term that describes when the blood's potassium levels are too low. Potassium is an important electrolyte that is responsible for healthy functioning of nerve and muscle cells - especially the muscle cells in the heart. The kidneys control the body's potassium levels including allowing excess potassium to leave the body through urine or sweat.

Insulin – Insulin is the name of a hormone that helps to regulate metabolism of fat and carbohydrates in the body.

Ki-67 – This term refers to a "biomarker[23]" used to measure the relative activity of a tumor.

Metastases - This term describes the spread of cancer cells from an original tumor site to various other parts of the body.

MRI - This is an acronym for "Magnetic Resonance Imaging." MRIs produce detailed images of the body through use of radio

---

[22] **Allergen** – An allergen is a substance that causes an allergic reaction.
[23] **Biomarker** – A "biomarker," or, "biological marker," generally refers to a measurable indicator of some biological state or condition. The term occasionally is also used to refer to a substance whose detection indicates the presence of a living organism.

MY JOURNEY WITH NEUROENDOCRINE CANCER
What You Don't Know Can Kill You!

waves and magnates. Use of a MRI is a valuable tool used by doctors to aid in the diagnosis of various conditions in the body.

Neuroendocrine Tumors (NETs) - Neuroendocrine tumors are a highly diverse group of tumors formed by neuroendocrine cells. Because neuroendocrine cells are found throughout the body, NETs can arise in a various organs including those of the gastrointestinal system, lungs, skin and thymus.

Neuroendocrine tumors release hormones into the blood in response to signals from the nervous system. Such release of hormones from NETs into the body often result in unpleasant, painful side effects. NET tumors may be benign (not cancerous) or they may, in fact, be malignant (cancerous).

Examples of neuroendocrine tumors are carcinoid tumors, islet cell tumors, Merkel cell cancer (carcinoma of the skin), medullary thyroid cancer, pheochromocytomas[24], neuroendocrine small cell lung cancer and large cell neuroendocrine carcinoma (a rare type of lung cancer).

Octreotide - Octreotide is an octapeptide[25] that mimics natural somatostatin pharmacologically, though it is a more potent inhibitor of growth hormone, glucagon and insulin than the natural hormone.

Octreo-Scan - This is the name of a scan that requires injection of a radioactive material, "octreotide" (see above), into a vein to allow subsequent display of tumor cells in the body that have somatostatin

---

[24] **Pheochromocytoma** - A "pheochromocytoma" is a rare adrenaline-producing tumor that arises from adrenal glands.
[25] **Octapeptide** – Octapeptide is a protein fragment or molecule (as oxytocin or vasopressin) that consists of eight amino acids linked in a polypeptide chain.

receptors.

Octreotide Acetate – This is a synthetic somatostatin that is able to inhibit excess hormones produced by various neuroendocrine tumors.

Pancreatic Carcinoid Tumor – This is type of carcinoid tumor is found on the pancreas. It is **NOT** the same as pancreatic cancer.

Pancreatic Enzyme – This is the name of a protein that is secreted in the pancreas. It aids in the digestion of food.

PICC – A "PICC" is a peripherally inserted Central Catheter, a thin, flexible tube inserted into a vein in the arm. It can be used for infusion treatments or to draw blood.

Port – A "port" is a small, round disc that attaches to a catheter placed just beneath the skin. It is usually placed in the chest or in the abdomen. The attached catheter is inserted into a vein for easier drug or fluid infusion.

Portal Vein – A "portal vein" is one that divides into the right and left branches in the liver. 75% of the blood circulation to the liver flows through the portal vein.

PRRT - This is an acronym for "Peptide Receptor Radionuclide Therapy" - a nuclear medicine therapy involving the systemic treatment of metastasized neuroendocrine tumors. The first patients were treated in 1996.

Radiofrequency Ablation – This is a form of heat treatment similar to cryoblation except that it uses heat rather than cold to kill tumors.

Sandostatin – This is the brand name for Octreotide Acetate that is manufactured by the Novartis Pharmaceutical Company.

Sandostatin LAR – This is a long-acting version of Octreotide Acetate given by depot injection.

Serotonin – This is a compound found in the brain, blood serum and gastric membranes. Levels of serotonin are often found to be elevated in carcinoid patients.

Sir Spheres – These are radioactive microspheres that emit Yttrium 90 (a radioactive isotope). Sir Spheres are injected directly into the hepatic artery.

Somatostatin Analogues – The term, Somatostatin Analogues, describes the manufactured versions of the hormone, somatostatin. These are designed to reduce the excessive secretion of hormones from carcinoid tumors and certain types of endocrine pancreatic tumors (glucagonoma, VIPoma and gastrinoma).

By so doing, Somatostatin Analogues have a lasting effect to reduce the painful, unpleasant symptoms caused by the over secretion (i.e. the syndrome) of somatostatin from neuroendocrine tumors. Current examples of Somatostatin Analogue today include Octreotide, (Sandostatin), Lanreotide (Somatuline) and Pasireotide.

Somatostatin Receptors (SSTRs) - Somatostatin Analogues bind to these receptors (or at least they try to). The subtypes expressed by NETs are variable and the efficiency of different Somatostatin Analogues to bind to each Somatostatin Receptor varies. Non-functional NETs have SSTRs and so Somatostatin Analogues will bind to them although less efficiently.

Somatostatin Receptor Scintigraphy - This is a type of radionuclide scan used to find carcinoid and other types of tumors. Radioactive octreotide, a drug similar to somatostatin, is injected into a vein and travels through the bloodstream.

The radioactive octreotide attaches to tumor cells that have receptors for somatostatin. A radiation-measuring device detects the radioactive octreotide, and makes pictures showing where the tumor cells are located in the body. This is also called an octreotide scan and SRS.

Subcutaneous – This is a term that refers to the area located just beneath the skin.

Theraspheres – This is a procedure that uses tiny glass beads to inject radiation directly into tumors using Yttrium90.

Tincture of Opium – This is an opiate that is used to slow chronic diarrhea which is often experienced by carcinoid patients.

TPN – This is an acronym for **T**otal **P**arental **N**utrition. TPN is often given to patients who are no longer able to digest food. TPN does not utilize the digestive system.

Tumor Debulking – This is a term that describes a surgical procedure for removing as much of an existing tumor as is possible.

VIP – This is an acronym for **V**asoactive **I**ntestinal **P**olypeptide. VIP is the primary peptide that is produced by the majority of pancreatic tumors ("VIPomas") causing WDHHA.

MY JOURNEY WITH NEUROENDOCRINE CANCER
What You Don't Know Can Kill You!

WDHHA – This is an acronym for **W**atery **D**iarrhea **H**ypokalemia, **H**ypochlorhydria and Acidosis.

BOB WALSH

MY JOURNEY WITH NEUROENDOCRINE CANCER
What You Don't Know Can Kill You!

EXHIBIT A

Letter Sent to Local Clergy Regarding Miraculous Disappearance of Two Deadly Tumors

Robert T. Walsh
162 Liberty Street, Deer Park, NY 11729

October 14, 2018

Most Reverend John O. Barres	Monsignor Robert J. Clerkin
Diocese of Rockville Centre	Ss. Cyril & Methodius
Rockville Centre, NY 11571-9023	Deer Park, NY 11729

Dear Bishop Barres and Monsignor Clerkin:

This letter confirms my recent phone message to each of you regarding a miraculous experience in which a deadly, cancerous tumor literally disappeared from my body ... not once ... but twice.

    The first time this happened was in late February 2017 soon after I was diagnosed with a rare, incurable malignancy, neuroendocrine (NET) cancer. During exploratory surgery at North Shore Hospital on Long Island, biopsies were taken of a tumor that had completely closed my digestive system leaving me in danger of dying. Pathologists at four different cancer centers (Lenox Hill Hospital, Montefiore Hospital, National Institutes of Health and St. Francis Hospital) later examined these biopsies and confirmed it was the rare, incurable neuroendocrine cancer.

    Family members, friends and rosary societies in St. Cyril and St. Matthew Churches joined me in praying for God's help. The doctor who first discovered the cancer went in a second time to cut away some of the tumor in an effort as he said, "to give you a little more time." As soon as the surgery was finished, the doctor came out and exclaimed, "It's gone; the tumor is gone!"

Subsequently, extensive tests at six other cancer centers showed the deadly tumor did inexplicably disappear without any chemo or surgery. Brilliant oncologists in cancer research centers studying this rare cancer could not explain how this could possibly have happened. As one stated, "I don't understand how such a tumor could simply disappear. This type of cancer roots itself deeply within the body ... like a tree roots itself in the ground."

For those oncologists who still doubted, God performed the very same miracle a second time! In August of this year, CT/PET and special MRI scans showed that the cancerous tumor had returned at the bottom of the common bile duct ... only this time it was much larger. Accordingly, on October 2, oncologists at Mount Sinai Cancer Center in New York City conducted exploratory surgery to determine what, if any, surgical alternatives might be done.

The results were precisely the same as the first time 18 months earlier ... all the biopsies taken showed the tumor had once again miraculously disappeared. The surgeon who previously said they were all looking for a scientific explanation called with results of the biopsies.

He stated, "We cannot understand what has happened; the tumor is gone. There is no scientific explanation other than it truly is miraculous!"

While everyone agreed the tumors "mysteriously" disappeared, they also confirmed I still have the NET cancer throughout my body. In fact, one of the worst remaining tumors in my body is located adjacent to my spine where they cannot safely get at it surgically. I suffer badly from the terrible effects of the cancer in my body but God gives me the strength to endure this while offering up my sufferings for the holy souls in Purgatory.

MY JOURNEY WITH NEUROENDOCRINE CANCER
What You Don't Know Can Kill You!

My wife, Margie, and I shared with all the oncologists studying me, that the miracle disappearance of the tumors was in response to many rosaries and Masses offered on my behalf. With no scientific evidence to show otherwise, these medical scientists have acknowledged the only plausible explanation for the disappearing tumors can only be miraculous.

I thought you both would be interested in hearing such wonderful news. I have attached copies of the operating, pathology and radiology reports that provide clear, indisputable scientific evidence of what happened – not once but twice. It is like God wanted to make sure we got the message that prayer, especially the greatest prayer of all – the Eucharist, really helps.

May God continue to bless you both for all you do in His Holy Name; I remain, sincerely,

Bob Walsh

Attachment: Copies of related operating, pathology and radiology reports evidencing miraculous disappearance of two deadly tumors

BOB WALSH

EXHIBIT B

Biopsy Pathology Report Shows 1st NET Tumor
North Shore Hospital - March 2, 2017

Northwell Health
Northwell Health Laboratories

NORTH SHORE UNIVERSITY HOSPITAL
300 COMMUNITY DRIVE, MANHASSET, NY 11030
(516) 304-7284 FAX (516) 304-7269

ANATOMIC PATHOLOGY SERVICES

Patient Name: WALSH, ROBERT T
Medical Record #: 001280523
DOB: 1/25/1945 Sex: Male
Location: MH END
Submitting Physician: BANSAL, RAJIV
Copy to Physician:

Accession #: 10- S-17-004107
Account #: 600003685242
Collection Date: 2/27/2017
Received Date: 2/27/2017

Surgical Pathology Report

Report Date: 3/2/2017 1:21:48 PM

Final Diagnosis

1. Ampulla, biopsy:
   - Well differentiated neuroendocrine neoplasm, grade 1, see note.

Note: Tissue is fragmented with marked cautery artifact. The tumor size, mitotic count, margin, lymphovascular invasion cannot be evaluated. Immunohistochemical stains for Chromogranin, Synaptophysin, and Ki-67 confirm the diagnosis. Dr. Fan has reviewed this part and concurred the diagnosis.

2. Stomach, antrum, biopsy:
   - Gastric antral type mucosa with intestinal metaplasia.
   - Negative for H. pylori (Warthin Starry stain).

Lihui Qin, M.D.
(Electronic Signature)
Reported on: 03/02/17

Clinical History
r/o CBD stone, dilated gallbladder, abdominal pain
Gastritis, r/o adenoma

Specimen(s) Submitted
1. Ampulla
2. Antrum biopsy

Gross Description
1. The specimen is received in formalin and the specimen container is labeled: **Ampulla biopsy**. It consists of six fragments of tan-pink soft tissue ranging from 0.1 cm to 0.3 cm in greatest dimension. Entirely submitted. One cassette

2. The specimen is received in formalin and the specimen container is labeled: **Antrum biopsy**. It consists

Patient: WALSH, ROBERT T
DISCH: 2/27/2017
Printed: 3/3/2017
Page 1 of 2

Physician: BANSAL, RAJIV
2001 MARCUS AVENUE
SUITE E130
LAKE SUCCESS, NY
11042

MY JOURNEY WITH NEUROENDOCRINE CANCER
What You Don't Know Can Kill You!

EXHIBIT C

Biopsy Pathology Report Shows 1st NET Disappeared!
Saint Francis Hospital – April 17, 2017

Saint Francis Hospital
100 Port Washington Blvd
Roslyn, NY 11576
Laboratory Director: Jeffrey A. Hamilton, M.D.
Phone Fax Number: 516-562-6410 516-562-6427
Ordering Physician: BANSAL, RAJIV
Consulting Physician:

Patient Name: WALSH, ROBERT
MRN: 2237290
DOB: 01/25/1943 Sex: Male
FIN: 17/0200522
Location: FEN, ENDO 02

7-SP-17-003074

Pathology Reports

Accession
7-SP-17-003074

Collected Date/Time
04/17/2017 14:46

Received Date/Time
04/17/2017 19:03

Surgical Pathology Report

Diagnosis

A. Ampulla, biopsy:
- Benign duodenal mucosa with non specific chronic inflammation. The villous architecture appears preserved. There is no evidence of neuroendocrine neoplasm.

B. Stomach, antrum, biopsy:
- Predominantly oxyntic type mucosa with chronic gastritis. Negative for active inflammation, intestinal metaplasia and neuroendocrine tumor. Modified Giemsa stain demonstrates possible luminal bacterial forms, negative for H. pylori by immunohistochemistry.

C. Stomach, body, biopsy:
- Mild non specific chronic gastritis. Negative for neuroendocrine tumor. Modified Giemsa stain for Helicobacter pylori is negative.

John C. Chumas, MD (Electronic Signature)
Reported: 04/20/17 08:24
JCC dv

Ancillary Studies
Immunohistochemistry (7SP17-3074 Block B1)

H. pylori: Negative

W. Liu, M.D.

Appropriate positive and negative tissue control slides for this immunohistochemical study have been reviewed and show expected staining patterns. The study utilizes Ventana ultraView detection system.

Technical component performed at Catholic Health Services Regional Laboratory, 70 Arkay Drive, Hauppauge, NY 11788
Professional component performed at Catholic Health Services Regional Laboratory, 70 Arkay Drive, Hauppauge, NY 11788

Clinical Information
Neuroendocrine tumor, ampulla lesion.

Patient: WALSH, ROBERT   Report Request ID: 40117638

BOB WALSH

EXHIBIT D

CT/PET Scan Report Shows 2nd NET Tumor
Northwell Health - August 27, 2018

NORTHWELL HEALTH

Northwell Imaging at Bay Shore

An Extension of Long Island Jewish Medical Center
440 E Main St., Suite D, Bay Shore, NY, 11706 631-414-8000 631-414-8039

Department of Radiology

HEAD/NECK: Unchanged nodule anterior margin left thyroid lobe extending into the isthmus, 1.8 x 1.8 cm and smaller nodule in the lower right thyroid lobe 1.4 x 1.4 cm (both seen on image 190). Physiologic radiotracer activity in pituitary gland, salivary glands, and thyroid gland.

THORAX: Physiologic radiotracer activity.

LUNGS: No abnormal radiotracer activity. No lung nodule.

PLEURA/PERICARDIUM: No pleural or pericardial effusion.

HEPATOBILIARY/PANCREAS: Physiologic activity. Liver SUV mean is 9.8, previously 9.5

SPLEEN: Physiologic activity. Normal in size.

ADRENAL GLANDS: Physiologic activity. No nodule.

KIDNEYS/URINARY BLADDER: Physiologic radiotracer excretion.

REPRODUCTIVE ORGANS: No abnormal radiotracer activity.

ABDOMINOPELVIC NODES: No enlarged or somatostatin receptor-bearing lymph node.

BOWEL/PERITONEUM/MESENTERY: Unchanged radiotracer accumulation in the region of the ampulla (SUV 19.1; image 178), previous SUV 14.9, which is difficult to difficult to delineate on CT and to separate from adjacent physiologic activity in the uncinate process of the pancreas. Unchanged sigmoid colon anastomosis

BONES/SOFT TISSUES: Degenerative changes in the spine. No abnormal radiotracer activity.

IMPRESSION:

Since gallium-68 DOTATATE PET/CT March 28, 2017:

1. Unchanged somatostatin receptor-bearing ampullary lesion, consistent with known neuroendocrine tumor.

2. No new somatostatin receptor bearing sites of disease.

3. Unchanged bilateral thyroid nodules. Consider further evaluation with thyroid ultrasound.

MY JOURNEY WITH NEUROENDOCRINE CANCER
What You Don't Know Can Kill You!

EXHIBIT E

Biopsy Pathology Report Shows 2nd NET Tumor Disappeared!
Mount Sinai Hospital – October 2, 2018

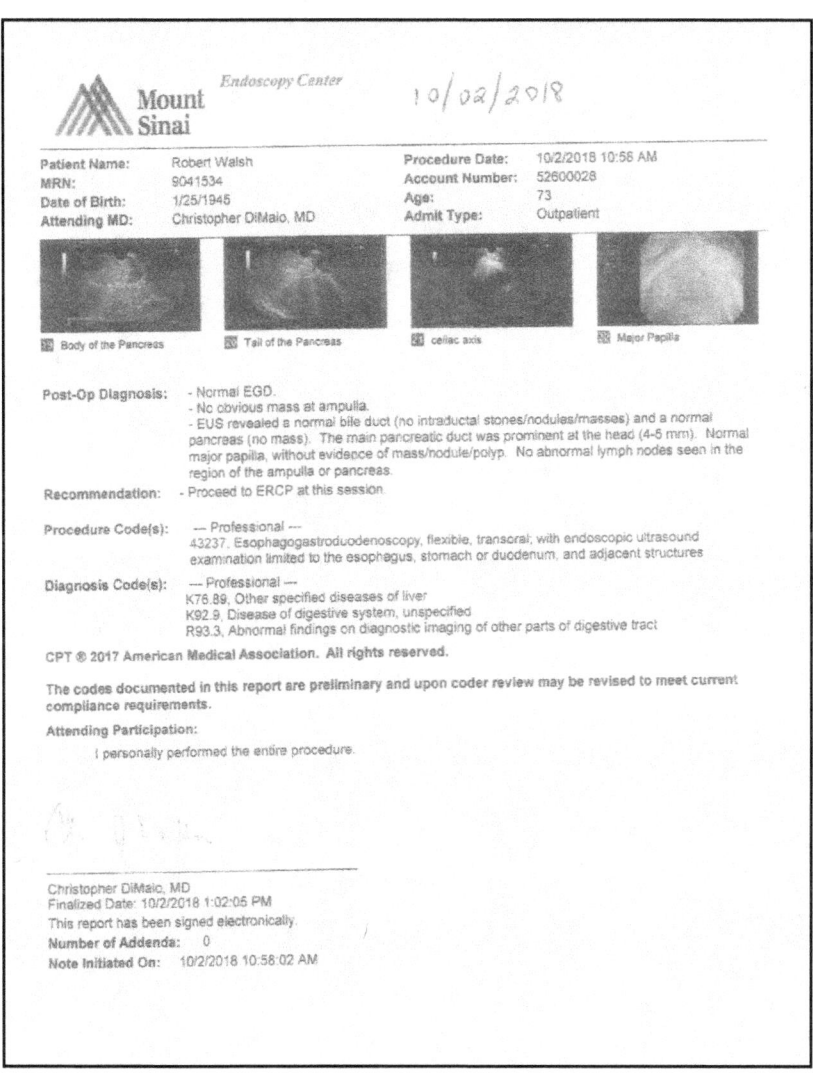

BOB WALSH

SELECT BOOKS
Published by PBJ Enterprises, Inc.

Available in paperback and eBook formats via www.Amazon.com.

INTERNATIONAL CAPITAL MARKETS
By Bob Walsh

This book is a practical guide on the operation of international capital markets and the ever present danger of money laundering. Topics include global banking, securities processing and global custody, regulatory compliance, technology systems and communications, and accounting. An important section includes the required components of an anti-money-laundering program.

THE DAY THEY KILLED JESUS CHRIST
By Bob Walsh

This book writes of the Passion of Jesus Christ as if the reader is actually present to witness the horrific, heart-breaking events as they unfolded. The graphic descriptions are based upon information as recorded in the Bible, Catholic Church teachings, studies of the Holy Shroud, visions by the saints and in reported ancient history.

HOW TERRORISTS MOVE MONEY THROUGH BANKS
Ways to Detect and Stop Terrorist Financing
By Bob Walsh

This book is a must for all banks seeking to detect and stop the illegal use of their services by terrorists and criminal organizations. A valuable guide is included for those working in anti-money laundering compliance. It provides critical information covering retail and institutional services and the many ways terrorists and criminal groups attempt to move dirty money through banks.

SELECT BOOKS
Published by PBJ Enterprises, Inc.
Available in paperback and eBook formats via www.Amazon.com.

MIRACLES AT SAINT ANNE'S SHRINE
At St. Jean the Baptiste Church in New York City
By Bob Walsh

This book describes several breath-taking miracles occurring at Saint Anne's Shrine in St. Jean the Baptiste Church in New York City. The events are based upon recorded ancient history, Catholic Church traditions and visions by the saints. Some of the miraculous events were personally witnessed by the author.

HISTORY OF THE GLOBAL SECURITIES INDUSTRY
By Bob Walsh

This book describes the global securities industry from ancient times to present day in terms of how this unique industry has evolved to make it possible for trillions of dollars a day in investment capital to move from one market to another, and from one country to another, all at lightning speed. Included is a discussion of market places, financial participant, services, currencies, securities, and applicable laws, rules and regulations.

MY LIFE OF MIRACLES
By Bob Walsh

This book shares miraculous experiences the author has personally witnessed over the course of his lifetime. He provides a first-hand account, a "peek behind the scenes," into the reality of God, the angels, the devil and the vast supernatural world surrounding us all.

SELECT BOOKS
Published by PBJ Enterprises, Inc.
Available in paperback and eBook formats via www.Amazon.com.

CONQUERING THE WILD WEST

EDITH KOHL'S HISTORIC BOOKS
Presented by her nephew, Cliff Ammons

RENOWNED AUTHOR - EDITH EUDORA AMMONS KOHL
Edith Eudora Ammons Kohl is one of the brave, talented women who helped settle America's wild, wild West. She truly is one of America's unsung heroines. Cliff Ammons, her nephew, now makes available for the first time ever, all four books written by Edith Kohl in which she captures the sights, sounds and exciting events as they happened. She wrote from her own personal experiences as she lived them! Her brilliant craft of words describes the grueling, sometimes tragic, harsh realities endured by so many of those involved in the taming of our country's wild, wild West. These historic books are a valuable treasure for all Americans who value the beginnings of our country.

LAND OF THE BURNT THIGH
One Woman's Conquest of the Wild, Wild West

THE SODBREAKERS
People Who Lived and Died Settling the West

WOMAN OF THE CAVALCADE
An Epic True Story

DENVER'S FIRST CHRISTMAS
A Unique, Historic Commentary

BOB WALSH

MY JOURNEY WITH NEUROENDOCRINE CANCER
What You Don't Know Can Kill You!

INDEX

5-HIAA, 142, 157, 191
AARP, 64, 70
Acromegaly, 165
Adrenal Glands, 191
AdrenoCorticotropic Hormone (ACTH), 152
Allergen, 194
Ampulla of Vater, 4, 12, 19, 20, 26, 27, 42, 45, 47, 48, 56, 61, 68, 99, 140, 141
Analogue, 57, 197
Angels, 210
Avastin Eye Medication, 8, 17, 50, 51
Bethesda, Maryland, 45, 46, 49, 53, 71, 87
Bile, 191
Biliary Tree, 3, 4, 20
Biomarker, 194
Blessed Mother, 30, 31, 32, 33
Bob Walsh, 209, 210
Butt Dart, 70
Carcinoid, 47, 58, 142, 147, 150, 164, 181, 183, 184, 189, 191
Carcinoid Crisis, 165, 191
Carcinoid Syndrome, 58, 140, 143, 152, 157, 160, 161, 163, 167, 192
Carcinoid Tumors, 147
Carcinoids, 147, 191
Carcinoma, 192
Catheter, 192, 196
Center for Carcinoid and Neuroendocrine Tumors, 107
Center for Eye Care, 8
Chemo-Embolization, 193
Chromogranin A, 144, 192
Cliff Ammons, 211
Columbia Hospital Cancer Center, 4
Computed Tomography, 55
Cryoblation, 192
CT, 55

CT/PET Scan, vi, 4, 31, 41, 55, 56, 123, 202, 206
Deer Park, Long Island, ix
Depot Injection, 192
Diana Walsh, vii, 43, 45, 46, 49, 53, 54, 55, 56, 57, 59, 60, 69, 71, 72, 73, 87, 91, 95, 96, 97, 111
Diarrhea, 155, 156, 158
Diuretic, 193
Divine Mercy, 2, 29
Dopamine, 193
Dr. Alan Mechanic, 113
Dr. Arnbjorn Toset, 117, 118
Dr. Da, 96, 97
Dr. Daniel Kohane, 105, 112, 115
Dr. David Fastenberg, 51
Dr. Dmitri Alden, 23, 24, 25, 26, 27, 28, 29, 36, 38, 40, 41
Dr. Edward M. Wolin, 43, 45, 107, 111
Dr. Gregory Persak, 7
Dr. Grossly Inept, v, 63, 64, 65, 66, 67, 69, 70, 77, 78, 83, 99, 105, 106, 107, 108, 109, 111, 112, 115
Dr. Howard Hertz, 1, 2, 3, 97, 98, 105, 115, 117
Dr. Jeremy L. Davis, 71
Dr. Kwekkeboom, 179, 180
Dr. Matthew Strachovsky, 8, 9, 15, 50, 51, 75, 81
Dr. Rajiv Bansal, 3, 4, 11, 12, 13, 19, 23, 47, 48, 49, 59, 61, 62, 79, 85
Dr. Richard Baum, 180
Dr. Robert Shamul, 49
Dr. Robert Turoff, 41
Dr. Stephen A. Wank, 54, 55, 56, 57, 58, 59, 62, 87, 96
Edith Ammons Kohl, 211
Edmond J. Safra, 53, 54
Endocrine Pancreatic Tumors, 197

Endocrine System, 193
Endoscope, 193
Endoscopic Retrograde Cholangio Pancreatography (ERCP), 5
Endoscopic Ultrasound (EUS), 5
Endoscopy, 5, 7, 11, 47, 49, 59, 62, 79, 85, 193
ERCP, 5, 11, 79, 123, 126, 129, 168
Eucharistic Minister, ix
EUS, 5, 11, 47, 79, 123, 126, 129
Eylea Eye Medication, 51, 52, 75, 81
F-Dopa, 55, 56, 61
Foregut Carcinoid Tumors, 152
Foregut Tumors, 157
Gallbladder, 4, 5, 11, 20, 26, 62, 69, 128, 159, 191
Gallium-68, 87
Gallium-68 Dotatate, 28, 41, 169
Garden of Gethsemane, 30
Gastrin, 144, 158, 193
Gastrinoma, 164, 197
Gastrinomas, 151
Glucagon, 193
Governor of New York, ix
Hemochromatosis, ix, 2, 83
Hepatic Artery, 193
Hindgut Carcinoid Tumors, 153
Histamine, 194
Holy Name Society, ix
Holy Sacrifice of the Mass, 133
Holy Shroud, 209
Hormones, 141, 157, 160, 194
Hypercalcemia, 158, 159
Hypertension, 23, 58, 62, 156, 160, 161
Hypokalemia, 158, 194
Immunohistochemical Staining, 144
Insulin, 194
Insulinomas, 151
Iodine, 87, 88, 89, 90, 91, 92, 93, 94, 95, 96, 97, 98, 117
Iohexol, 91, 92, 93
Ipsen Pharmaceuticals, 142
Irritable Bowel Syndrome (IBS), 156
Jesus Christ, 209
Joanne Forbes, P.A., 49, 55
Ki-67, 194
Knights of Columbus, ix
Lake Success, Long Island, 3, 61
Land of the Burnt Thigh, 211
Lanreotide, 61, 69, 142, 143, 197
Lenox Hill Hospital, 24
LI Vitroretinal, 51
Liver, 2, 3, 4, 5, 11, 20, 128, 147, 149, 155, 167, 170, 171, 176, 177, 178, 191, 192, 193, 196
Luke, 135
Lumen Barium, 87
Manhasset, Long Island, 11, 79
Margie Holly Walsh, iii, vii, ix, x, 1, 3, 5, 9, 12, 13, 24, 26, 27, 28, 29, 30, 35, 36, 37, 38, 39, 40, 42, 48, 61, 64, 67, 71, 72, 73, 77, 78, 79, 105, 111, 115, 122, 125, 126, 127, 128, 129, 203
Mass, 136
Matthew, 135
Medicare, 64, 70
Metastases, 194
Midgut Carcinoid, 157
Midgut Carcinoid Tumors, 152
Monsignor Dominic Ashkar, 59, 72
Montefiore Einstein Center for Cancer Care, 43, 107
Mount Sinai Hospital, 41, 107, 109
MRCP, 2, 3, 4, 121
MRI, 2, 23, 55, 56, 105, 115, 194
National Cancer Institute, 139, 150, 186
National Institutes of Health, v, 45, 46, 49, 50, 53, 54, 55, 56, 59, 61, 62, 68, 69, 71, 72, 73, 87, 90, 91, 92, 93, 94, 95, 96, 97, 98, 117, 139, 186, 189
Naturopathic Medicine, 173
NET cancer, 155, 181, 183, 186,

187
NETs, 139, 141, 142, 143, 147, 183, 197
neuroendocrine, 42, 137, 138, 139, 181, 183, 184, 187, 192, 195, 196
Neuroendocrine Cancer, iii, vii, ix, x, xi, xv, xvi, 20, 23, 24, 25, 26, 30, 33, 35, 36, 37, 38, 39, 40, 41, 42, 43, 45, 46, 47, 50, 51, 52, 54, 55, 58, 59, 60, 61, 62, 63, 65, 66, 67, 68, 69, 71, 75, 77, 78, 79, 83, 85, 86, 87, 91, 100, 107, 109, 111, 112, 117, 118, 119, 121, 122, 124, 125, 126, 127, 129, 133, 137, 139, 140, 141, 142, 144, 148, 149, 165, 167, 170, 171, 172, 173, 177, 179, 191, 192, 201
Neuroendocrine Tumor, 20, 36, 38, 41, 42, 45, 47, 48, 49, 55, 56, 57, 61, 68, 72, 85, 122, 123, 128, 129, 140, 141, 143, 144, 155, 160, 164, 171, 175, 186
Neuroendocrine Tumor Research Foundation, 178
Neuroendocrine Tumors, 55, 56, 58, 71, 112, 143, 145, 147, 149, 150, 167, 168, 175, 176, 180, 183, 184, 195, 196, 197
Neurotransmitters, 137
New York City, ix, 24, 29, 32, 36, 41, 210
NIH Catholic Chaplain, 59
North Shore Hospital, 3, 11, 19, 23, 79, 85, 124, 125, 201, 204
Northwell Imaging Laboratory, 41
Northwell Laboratories, 40
Novartis Pharmaceutical, 66, 67, 108, 109, 142, 187, 197
Octapeptide, 195
Octreo-Scan, 195
Octreotide, 71, 72, 127, 142, 176, 180, 195, 196, 197
Octreotide Acetate, 196
Pancreas, 2, 3, 4, 5, 11, 20, 26, 128, 129, 139, 147, 149, 150, 152, 175, 192, 193, 196
Pancreatic Carcinoid Tumor, 196
Pancreatic Enzyme, 196
Pasireotide, 197
Patrick Victor Walsh, 59
PBJ Enterprises, Inc., iii, 209, 210, 211
Peggie Murano Fabian, 12, 13, 48, 79
Peptides, 157, 160
Periampullary Cancer, 5
Periampullary Lesion, 3
PICC, 196
Pietrelcina, Italy, 7
pNETS, 151
Port, 196
Portal Vein, 196
PPomas, 151
PRRT (Peptide Receptor Radionuclide Therapy), 175, 176, 177, 178, 179, 180, 196
Purgatory, 7, 14, 49, 51, 81, 117, 202
Pyx, 60
Radiofrequency Ablation, 196
Russia, ix
Safra Lodge, 54
Saint Anne, 30, 31, 32, 33, 210
Saint Anne's Shrine, 28, 29, 31, 36
Saint Anne's Shrine, 29, 210
Saint Faustina Kowalska, 3
Sandostatin, 61, 65, 66, 67, 69, 70, 77, 78, 83, 84, 99, 107, 108, 109, 111, 112, 113, 115, 142, 143, 177, 197
Serotonin, 140, 142, 143, 144, 152, 153, 158, 165, 191, 192, 197
Sir Spheres, 197
Sloan Kettering, 31
Somatostatin, 58, 61, 62, 69, 141, 142, 143, 156, 195, 196, 197, 198
Somatostatin Analogues, 143, 197
Somatostatin Receptor

Scintigraphy, 198
Somatostatin Receptors, 143, 169, 176
Somatuline, 142, 197
Ss. Cyril and Methodius, ix
St. Elizabeth Catholic Church, v, 85
St. Francis Hospital, 47
St. Jean the Baptiste Church, 28, 29, 32, 210
St. Padre Pio, 7
St. Peter, xvi, 9, 17
Subcutaneous, 198
Substance P, 144, 158
The Sodbreakers, 211
Theraspheres, 198
Tincture of Opium, 198
TNM Staging System, 167
Total Parental Nutrition, 198
TPN, 198
Tumor Debulking, 198
Type 1 Gastric Carcinoid Tumors, 151
Type 2 Gastric Carcinoid Tumors, 151
Type 3 Gastric Carcinoid Tumors, 152
U.S. Congress, ix
U.S. Goodwill Ambassador, ix
Ukraine, ix
Vasoactive Intestinal Polypeptide, 158, 198
VIP, 158, 159, 160, 198
VIPoma, 150, 197
Wall Street, ix, 68
Washington D.C., 5
WDHHA, 158, 159, 160, 198, 199
West Islip, Long Island, 8, 81
Wet Macular Degeneration, 8, 15, 16, 50, 51, 75, 81
Whipple Surgery, 23, 27, 28, 31, 38, 41, 47
Woman of the Cavalcade, 211
X-rays, 25, 55
Yorkville, ix
Zebra, 20, 21, 149
Zollinger-Ellison (ZE) Syndrome, 151, 158, 159, 160
Zwanger-Pesiri Radiology, 2, 3, 40, 98

MY JOURNEY WITH NEUROENDOCRINE CANCER
What You Don't Know Can Kill You!

NOTES

BOB WALSH

NOTES

MY JOURNEY WITH NEUROENDOCRINE CANCER
What You Don't Know Can Kill You!

NOTES

BOB WALSH

NOTES

MY JOURNEY WITH NEUROENDOCRINE CANCER
What You Don't Know Can Kill You!

NOTES

BOB WALSH

NOTES